RENAL DISEASE
Classification and Atlas of Tubulo-Interstitial Diseases

Prepared by the World Health Organization
Collaborating Centre for the Histological Classification
of Renal Diseases

Jacob Churg   **Ramzi S. Cotran**

Raja Sinniah   **Hiroshi Sakaguchi**

Leslie H. Sobin

and pathologists and nephrologists in 17 countries

IGAKU-SHOIN   **Tokyo • New York**

Published and distributed by
IGAKU-SHOIN Ltd.,
    5-24-3 Hongo, Bunkyo-ku, Tokyo
IGAKU-SHOIN Medical Publishers, Inc.,
    1140 Avenue of the Americas, New York, N.Y. 10036

Library of Congress Cataloging in Publication Data

Main entry under title:
Renal disease.
    Includes bibliographies and index.
    1. Nephritis, Interstitial—Classification.
2. Nephritis, Interstitial—Atlases.   3. Kidney
tubules—Diseases—Classification.   4. Kidney
tubules—Diseases—Atlases.   I. Churg, Jacob, 1910-
II. World Health Organization. Collaborating Centre
for Histological Classification of Renal Diseases.
[DNLM: 1. Kidney Diseases—classification—atlases.
2. Nephritis, Interstitial—classification—atlases.
WJ 17 R393]
RC918.N37R46   1984   616.6′1   84-9118
ISBN: 0-89640-104-9 (New York)
ISBN: 4-260-14104-X (Japan)

Printed and bound in Japan
10 9 8 7 6 5 4 3 2 1

World Health Organization Collaborating Centre for the Histological Classification of Renal Diseases, Department of Pathology, Mount Sinai School of Medicine, New York, N.Y., USA

Dr. Jacob Churg, Head of the Collaborating Centre.

Subcommittee on Tubulo-Interstitial Renal Diseases:

Dr. G. Andres, Department of Pathology, State University of New York at Buffalo, Buffalo, New York, USA.

Dr. A. W. Asscher, KRUF Institute of Renal Disease. Royal Infirmary, Cardiff, Wales, United Kingdom.

Dr. G. G. Avtandilov, Ministerstvo Sdravochranenia SSSR, Moscow, USSR.

Dr. A. Bergstrand, Department of Pathology, Huddinge Hospital, Huddinge, Sweden.

Dr. R. Cotran (Chairman), Department of Pathology, Brigham and Women's Hospital, Boston, Massachusetts, USA.

Dr. F. J. Gloor, Institut für Pathologie, Kantonsspital, St. Gallen, Switzerland.

Dr. G. Richet, Service de Nephrologie, Hopital Tenon, Paris, France.

Dr. R. A. Risdon, Department of Morbid Anatomy, Institute of Pathology, The London Hospital, London, England.

Dr. H. Sakaguchi, Department of Pathology, School of Medicine, Keio University, Tokyo, Japan.

Dr. R. Sinniah (Secretary), Department of Pathology, University of Singapore, Sepoy Lines, Singapore.

Dr. W. Thoenes, Pathologisches Institut der Universität Mainz, Mainz, Federal Republic of Germany.

Subcommittee on Vascular Renal Diseases:

Dr. E. L. Becker, Department of Medicine, Beth Israel Medical Center, New York, N.Y., USA.

Dr. R. H. Heptinstall (Chairman), Department of Pathology, The Johns Hopkins Hospital, Baltimore, Maryland, USA.

Dr. J. Hoedemaeker, Department of Pathology, State University of Leiden, Leiden, The Netherlands.

Dr. P. Kincaid-Smith, Department of Nephrology, Royal Melbourne Hospital, Parkville, Victoria, Australia.

Dr. S. Olsen (Secretary), University Institute of Pathology, Aarhus Kommunehospital, Aarhus, Denmark.

Dr. L. Salinas-Madrigal, Department of Pathology, Instituto Nacional de Cardiologia, Mexico D.F., Mexico.

Dr. F. Skjorten, Patologisk anatomisk lab, Ulleval Sykehus, Oslo, Norway.

Dr. T. Tallqvist, Department of Pathology, Maria Hospital, Helsinki, Finland.

Acknowledgments

Most of the illustrations in this monograph were supplied by the members of the Collaborating Centre. Some illustrations came from friends and colleagues whose contributions are gratefully acknowledged: Doctors R. Adlersberg, H-S. Altman, R. Bulger, A. Y. Campbell, A. M. Churg, A. Cohen, R. Colvin, F. Dallenbach, I. Damjanov, G. Dammin, S. H. Dikman, R. S. Dobrin, J. L. Duffy, M. Elkin, T. Farragiana, M. Garrido, B. Gold, R. Goyer, E. Grishman, G. R. Hennigar, J. Hestbech, M. Hughson, D. B. Jones, S. M. Katz, A. F. Madrazo, M. Mellins, H-A. Muller, M. Needle, N. Pervez, A. Pheterson, C. L. Pirani, H. Rennke, S. Ribot, M. M. Schwartz, H. Sobel, K. Solez, B. H. Spargo, L. Strauss, R. K. Sibley, Y. Suzuki, C. Tisher, V. Totovic, E. Vazquez Martul, M. Venkatachalam, V. S. Venkataseshan, R. L. Vernier, R. Waldherr, R. Wedeen, W. Wegmann, I. Weiss and G. Yelin, and the International Study of Kidney Disease in Children. If any contributor's name has been inadvertently omitted, our gratitude is no less sincere.

Some of the illustrations are reproduced from books and journals with permission of the publishers and the authors:
American Journal of Anatomy and *Alan R. Liss, Inc.*: Figs. 1 and 10, Reference: Bulger and Nagle—Chapter 2. *Marcel Dekker, Inc.*: Fig. 2, Chapter 27, Reference: Solez and Whelton-Textbooks and Monographs. *International Academy of Pathology* and *The Williams and Wilkins Company*: Fig. 1, Chapter 8, Reference: Goyer—Chapter 9. *Kidney International*: Fig. 2, Reference: Hestbech et al.—Chapter 5. *Little, Brown and Company*: Fig. 1-36 and 1-37, Reference: Bulger—Chapter 2. *New England Journal of Medicine*: Figs. 4 and 5, Reference: Case Records of Massachusetts General Hospital (Colvin)—Chapter 4. *Pathology Annual* and *Appleton-Century-Crofts*: Fig. 17, Reference: Damjanov and Katz—Chapter 4. *W. B. Saunders Company*: Figs. 6-9, 6-24, 6-27 and 6-42, Reference: Asscher et al.—Textbooks and Monographs; Fig. 1-33, Reference: Tisher—Chapter 2; Figs. 29-5 and 29-9, Reference: Brenner and Rector—Textbooks and Monographs; Fig. 2-32, Reference: Chapman et al.—Chapter 2. *John Wiley and Sons, Inc.*: Figs. 53, 71 and 72—Chapter 5, Reference: Churg, et al.—Chapter 11.

Appreciation is also expressed to all the technical personnel, especially Mr. A. Prado and Mr. N. Katz.

Contents

		Page
Preface		x
Chapter 1.	Introduction and Classification of Tubulo-interstitial Diseases	1
Chapter 2.	Normal Tubule and Normal Interstitium	5
Chapter 3.	Infection: Acute and Chronic Pyelonephritis	21
	Acute Infectious Tubulo-interstitial Nephritis (acute pyelonephritis)	21
	Acute Bacterial Tubulo-interstitial Nephritis	21
	Fungal Tubulo-interstitial Nephritis	22
	Viral Tubulo-interstitial Nephritis	22
	Acute Tubulo-interstitial Nephritis Associated with Systemic Infection	22
	Chronic Infectious Tubulo-interstitial Nephritis (chronic pyelonephritis)	23
	Nonobstructive Reflux-Associated Chronic Pyelonephritis	23
	Vesicoureteral Reflex and Intrarenal Reflux	23
	Reflux Nephropathy	23
	Other Variants	25
	Chronic Obstructive Pyelonephritis Associated with Urinary Tract Obstruction	25
Chapter 4.	Infection: Special Forms of Pyelonephritis	34
	Xanthogranulomatous Pyelonephritis	34
	Malacoplakia	34
	Megalocytic Interstitial Nephritis	35
	Specific Renal Infections	35
	Tuberculosis	35
	Leprosy	35
	Syphilis	36
	Epidemic Hemorrhagic Fever	36
Chapter 5.	Drug-Induced Tubulo-interstitial Nephritis	55
	Acute Tubulotoxic Injury	55
	Drug-Induced Hypersensitivity Tubulo-interstitial Nephritis	55
	Chronic Drug-Induced Tubulo-interstitial Nephritis	56
	Analgesic Nephropathy	56
	Lithium Nephropathy	57
	Chloroethyl-cyclohexyl Nitrosourea (CCNU) Nephropathy	58

Chapter 6. Tubulo-interstitial Nephritis Associated with Immune
Disorders 77
    Tubulo-interstitial Nephritis Induced by Antibodies Re-
    acting with Tubular Antigens (antitubular basement mem-
    brane disease).. 77
        Antiglomerular Basement Membrane Glomerulone-
        phritis (Goodpasture's syndrome) 78
        Immune Complex Glomerulonephritis 78
        Drug Induced... 78
        Idiopathic.. 78
        Renal Allografts.. 78
    Tubulo-interstitial Nephritis Induced by Autologous or
    Exogenous Antigen-Antibody (immune) Complexes 79
        Systemic Lupus Erythematosus........................ 79
        Mixed Cryoglobulinemia 79
        Bacterial Immune Complex Glomerulonephritis 79
        Sjögren's Syndrome 79
        Hypocomplementemic Glomerulonephritis............ 80
        Renal Allografts.. 80
    Tubulo-interstitial Changes in Renal Allografts 80
    Tubulo-interstitial Nephritis Induced by, or Associated with,
    Cell-Mediated Hypersensitivity 81
    Tubulo-interstitial Nephritis Induced by Immediate (IgE-
    Type) Hypersensitivity................................... 82
Chapter 7. Obstructive Uropathy and Reflux Nephropathy............. 93
    Obstructive Uropathy.................................... 93
    Vesicoureteral Reflux Associated Nephropathy (reflux
    nephropathy) 94
Chapter 8. Tubulo-interstitial Nephritis Associated with Papillary
Necrosis 108
    Diabetes Mellitus 108
    Obstructive Uropathy.................................... 108
    Analgesic Nephropathy.................................. 108
    Hemorrhagic Necrosis of Papillae in the Newborn 109
Chapter 9. Heavy Metal-Induced Tubular and Tubulo-interstitial
Lesions 118
    Lead Nephropathy....................................... 118
    Mercury Nephropathy 119

Cisplatin Nephropathy.................................... 119

Cadmium Nephropathy.................................... 120

Other Heavy Metal-Induced Nephropathies.............. 120

    Gold Nephropathy 120

    Silver Nephropathy................................ 121

    Copper Nephropathy 121

    Iron Nephropathy 121

Chapter 10. Acute Tubular Injury/Necrosis 136

    Nephrotoxic Acute Tubular Necrosis 137

    Ischemic Acute Tubular Necrosis (acute vasomotor

    nephropathy) 138

    Imcompatible Blood Transfusion 139

    Myoglobinuria 139

Chapter 11. Tubular and Tubulo-interstitial Nephropathy Caused by Met-

abolic Disturbances 157

    Hypercalcemic Nephropathy............................ 157

    Urate Nephropathy 158

    Oxalate Nephropathy 159

    Cystinosis 160

    Hypokalemic Nephropathy 160

Chapter 12. Hereditary Renal Tubulo-interstitial Disorders............ 184

    Hereditary Renal Tubulo-interstitial Disorders.......... 184

    Tubulo-interstitial Nephritis Associated with Neoplastic

    Disorders 184

    Plasma Cell Dyscrasias 184

      Myeloma Kidney.................................. 184

      Light-Chain Nephropathy.......................... 185

    Mixed IgG-IgM Cryoglobulinemia 186

    Waldenström's Macroglobulinemia.................... 186

    Leukemic and Lymphomatous Infiltration 187

Chapter 13. Tubulo-interstitial Lesions in Glomerular and Vascular

Diseases 192

    Acute and Chronic Glomerular Diseases 192

    Advanced Sclerosing Glomerular Diseases 192

    Ischemic Atrophy.................................... 193

    End-stage Kidney.................................... 193

Chapter 14. Miscellaneous Disorders........................ 199

    Radiation Nephritis.................................. 199

    Balkan Endemic Nephropathy.......................... 199

    Granulomatous Sarcoid Nephropathy 200

Tubulo-interstitial Nephritis of Unknown Etiologic Basis
(idiopathic) 200
    Acute Idiopathic Tubulo-interstitial Nephritis.......... 200
    Idiopathic Granulomatous Tubulo-interstitial Nephritis 201
    Chronic Idiopathic Tubulo-interstitial Nephritis........ 201
References... 209
Index 215

Preface

This monograph is the second in the series entitled Classification and Atlas of Renal Diseases. The first volume, Classification and Atlas of Glomerular Diseases was published in 1982. The current volume presents Classification and Atlas of Tubulo-Interstitial Disorders. As before, it represents a collaborative effort of pathologists and nephrologists from many countries of the world, and it is supported by the World Health Organization. The third volume, now in publication, will deal with Vascular Diseases of the Kidney and with Developmental and Hereditary Diseases. Classification of Tumours of the Kidney was published by WHO in 1981* and is not considered part of the present series.

The format of the current volume is similar to that previously employed. In the first chapter a Table of Classification is introduced based upon the information in the current literature and upon the personal experiences of the Committee members. Subsequent chapters deal with individual topics listed in the Classification Table, each providing a brief discussion of the clinical and pathologic findings, illustrations of the gross and microscopic features, and where appropriate, immunofluorescence pictures, electron micrographs and x-rays. The volume is concluded by a brief list of current references and a subject index.

---

* International Histological Classification of Tumours No 25: Histological Typing of Kidney Tumours, by F.K. Mostofi in collaboration with I.E. Sesterhenn, L.H. Sobin and pathologists in seven countries.

Key to Abbreviations

ATN	acute tubular necrosis
ARF	acute renal failure
BUN	blood urea nitrogen
Cis-Platin	cis-dichlorodiamine platinum II (p. 63)
GBM	glomerular basement membrane
H & E	hematoxylin and eosin
IC	immune complex
IRR	intrarenal reflux
PAS	periodic acid-Schiff's reagent
RBC	red blood cell
SLE	systemic lupus erythematosus
TBM	tubular basement membrane
TIN	tubulo-interstitial nephritis
VUR	vesicoureteral reflux

CHAPTER 1

Introduction and Classification of Tubulo-interstitial Diseases

Introduction and Classification of Tubulo-interstitial Diseases

Tubulo-interstitial diseases are a diverse group of renal disorders in which the predominant morphologic changes occur in the tubules and interstitium. A great variety of etiologic agents and several pathogenetic mechanisms lead to tubulo-interstitial injury with similar histologic alterations; thus, a purely histologic classification of this group of disorders is inappropriate. For this reason, the suggested classification is one that takes into account etiologic, pathogenetic and clinical features.

Several points and reservations can be made with regard to this classification:

1. The terms *interstitial* and *tubulo-interstitial* are used interchangeably. Although it might be useful to distinguish between diseases that appear to start or predominate in the interstitium and those that involve mostly the tubules, in most instances interstitial and tubular lesions coexist, and even in experimental models, it often is difficult to pinpoint stages at which interstitial injury is isolated. In this book, the terms *nephritis* and *nephropathy* are used interchangeably.

2. Diseases are classified as acute or chronic, principally to enable recognition on the basis of clinicopathologic features. It sometimes is difficult to recognize acute interstitial disease on the basis of histologic criteria, particularly when it occurs on a background of focal or diffuse chronic renal disease. The infiltrate in acute interstitial diseases often is of the "chronic" type, with mononuclear cells predominating. Further, use of the terms *acute* and *chronic* disregards the fact that subacute, or healing, forms exist; an example is the healing phase of pyelonephritis. The classification outlined below is one in which the distinction between acute and chronic becomes unimportant and all such diseases can be combined under a single heading.

3. Although the various diseases are classified on the basis of a single etiologic agent in each case, in many instances the renal dysfunction in patients with serious chronic tubulo-interstitial diseases is due to more than one etiologic agent. For example, patients with vesicoureteral reflux may have infection and obstruction, and patients with urate nephropathy may have renal insufficiency as a result of exposure to lead.

4. The lack of glomerular involvement in the categorization of these disorders is inaccurate. On the one hand, tubulo-interstitial nephritis can be a component of primary and systemic glomerulonephritis and, on the other, it is now well recognized that glomerulosclerosis with proteinuria may be an important complication of tubulo-interstitial diseases, such as reflux nephropathy and analgesic nephropathy. These glomerular changes are discussed in the appropriate sections.

Table I Classification of Tubulo-interstitial
Diseases

Infection
  Acute Infectious Tubulo-interstitial Nephritis
    (acute pyelonephritis)
    Acute bacterial
    Fungal
    Viral
  Acute Tubulo-interstitial Nephritis Associated
    with Systemic Infection
    Group A streptococcal infection
    Diphtheria
    Toxoplasmosis
    Legionnaire's disease
    Brucellosis
    Viral infection
    Other variants
  Chronic Infectious Tubulo-interstitial Nephritis
    (chronic pyelonephritis)
    Nonobstructive reflux-associated chronic pye-
      lonephritis
    Other variants
    Chronic obstructive pyelonephritis
    Xanthogranulomatous pyelonephritis
    Malacoplakia
    Megalocytic interstitial nephritis
  Specific Renal Infections
    Tuberculosis
    Leprosy
    Syphilis
    Epidemic hemorrhagic fever
    Other variants
Drug-Induced Tubulo-interstitial Nephritis
  Acute Drug-Induced Tubulotoxic Injury
    Direct
    Indirect
  Drug-Induced Hypersensitivity Tubulo-intersti-
    tial Nephritis
  Chronic Drug-Induced Tubulo-interstitial Ne-
    phritis
    Analgesic nephropathy
    Lithium nephropathy
    Other (e.g., chloroethyl-cyclohexyl nitrosou-
      rea)
Tubulo-interstitial Nephritis Associated with Im-
  mune Disorders
  Induced by Antibodies Reacting with Tubular
    Antigens

Antiglomerular basement membrane glomer-
  ulonephritis or Goodpasture's syndrome
Immune complex glomerulonephritis
  Drugs
  Idiopathic
  Renal allografts
Induced by Autologous or Exogenous Antigen-
  Antibody Complexes
  Systemic lupus erythematosus
  Mixed cryoglobulinemia
  Bacterial immune complex glomerulonephri-
    tis
  Sjögren's syndrome
  Hypocomplementemic glomerulonephritis with
    vasculitis
  Renal allografts
Induced by, or associated with, cell-mediated
  hypersensitivity
  Bacterial, viral, or parasitic infection, drugs,
    chemicals
Induced by immediate (IgE-type) hypersensitiv-
  ity
  Drugs, parasitic infection(?)
Obstructive Uropathy
  Without infection (hydronephrosis)
  With infection
  Pyonephrosis
Vesicoureteral Reflux-Associated Nephropathy
  (reflux nephropathy)
Tubulo-interstitial Nephritis Associated with Pap-
  illary Necrosis
  Diabetes mellitus
  Obstructive uropathy
  Analgesic nephropathy
  Sickle cell disease nephropathy
  Hemorrhagic necrosis of papillae in the newborn
  Other variants (e.g., vascular disease, tubercu-
    losis)
Heavy Metal-Induced Tubular and Tubulo-inter-
  stitial Lesions
  Lead nephropathy
  Mercury nephropathy
  Cisplatin nephropathy
  Cadmium nephropathy
  Nephropathy induced by other heavy metals
    (gold, silver, copper, iron)

Table I (Continued)

Acute Tubular Injury/Necrosis
  Toxic
  Ischemic
  Severe crushing injury
  Abortion
  Extensive burn injury
  Shock
  Septicemia
  Other variants
  Incompatible blood transfusion
  Myoglobinuria
Tubular and Tubulo-interstitial Nephropathy Caused by Metabolic Disturbances
  Hypercalcemic nephropathy
  Urate nephropathy
  Oxalate nephropathy
  Cystinosis
  Hypokalemic nephropathy
  Vacuolar change (osmotic nephropathy)
  Glycogen deposition (as in glycogenosis or diabetes mellitus)
  Fatty changes
  Hyaline droplet degeneration
  Bile pigment deposition (bile nephrosis)
  Copper deposition (Wilson's disease)
  Iron deposition
Hereditary Renal Tubulo-interstitial Disorders
  Medullary cystic disease (juvenile nephron-ophthisis)

Familial interstitial nephritis of unknown etiologic basis
Alport's syndrome
Tubulo-interstitial Nephritis Associated with Neoplastic Disorders
  Plasma Cell Dyscrasias
    Myeloma kidney
    Light-chain nephropathy
  Mixed IgG-IgM cryoglobulinemia
  Waldenström's macroglobulinemia
  Leukemic and lymphomatous infiltration
Tubulo-interstitial Lesions in Glomerular and Vascular Diseases
  Acute and chronic glomerular diseases
  Ischemic atrophy
  End-stage kidney
Miscellaneous Disorders
  Radiation nephritis
  Balkan endemic nephropathy
  Granulomatous sarcoid nephropathy
  Tubulo-interstitial nephritis of unknown etiologic basis (idiopathic)
    Acute idiopathic tubulo-interstitial nephritis
    Idiopathic granulomatous tubulo-interstitial nephritis
    Chronic idiopathic tubulo-interstitial nephritis

CHAPTER 2

Normal Tubule and Normal Interstitium

Normal Tubule and Normal Interstitium

As is well known, the structure (and function) of the tubular cells varies along the length of a nephron from segment to segment and even within a segment. Detailed descriptions of each segment and its subdivisions, from the proximal tubule to the collecting duct, are given in standard textbooks of histology and in most textbooks of nephrology and nephropathology. In this atlas, illustrations are provided of the cells encountered in the proximal tubule, loop of Henle, distal tubule and collecting tubule and duct, together with a brief description of their salient features. This is meant to serve as a basis for comparison with the abnormal structure in disease. A similar approach is taken in regard to the renal interstitium. Its structure and cells are illustrated, and a brief description is given in the appropriate legends to figures.

Normal Tubule and Interstitium

Fig. 2-1   Thin (1 μm) section of renal cortex showing tubules and interstitium. Proximal tubules are characterized by intensely stained cytoplasm and high layer of brush border. (toluidine blue, ×300)

Fig. 2-2   Proximal tubules and renal interstitium. Brush border, elongated mitochondria and basal infoldings are visible. Interstitial space contains capillaries and interstitial cells (fibroblasts) with long processes. (electron micrograph, ×3000)

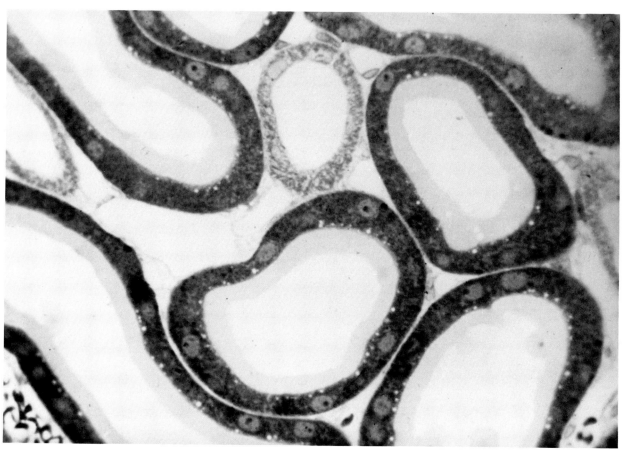
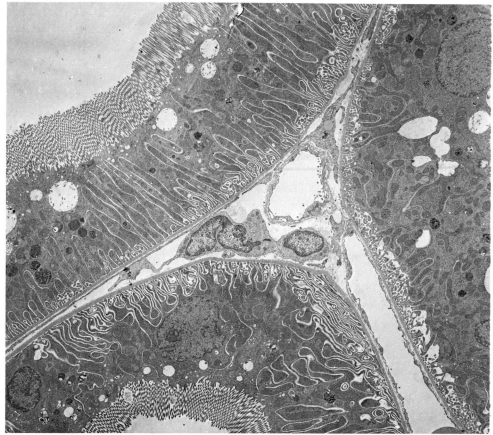

Normal Tubule and Interstitium

Fig. 2-3   Higher magnification of normal human proximal tubules (pars convoluta). Well-developed brush border lines the tubular lumen (at top of picture). Beneath the brush border are many apical vesicles and apical vacuoles. There are numerous mitochondria, which often are elongated. (electron micrograph, ×17,000)

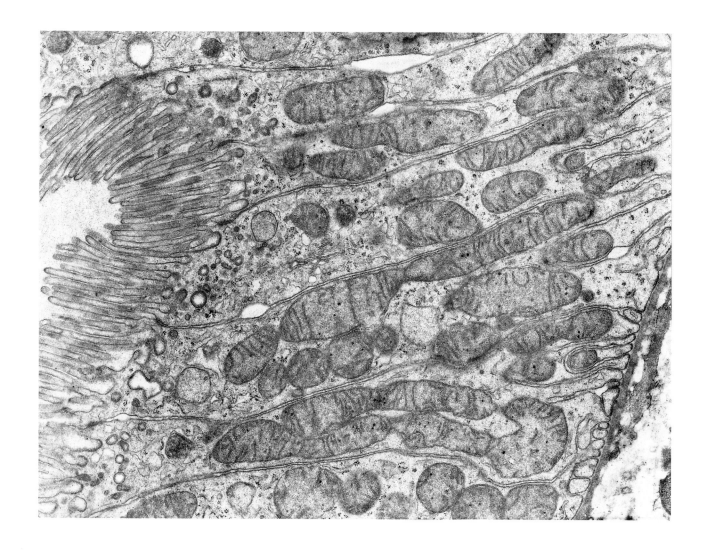

Normal Tubule and Interstitium

Fig. 2-4   Cross section of rabbit proximal tubule showing lumen, microvilli forming brush border and scattered cilia. At the base of the microvilli are apical vesicles. Lateral processes and basement membrane also are visible. (scanning electron micrograph, ×3000)

Fig. 2-5   Higher magnification of rabbit proximal convoluted tubule showing lateral processes in center, microvilli on right and basement membrane on left. (scanning electron micrograph, ×10,000)

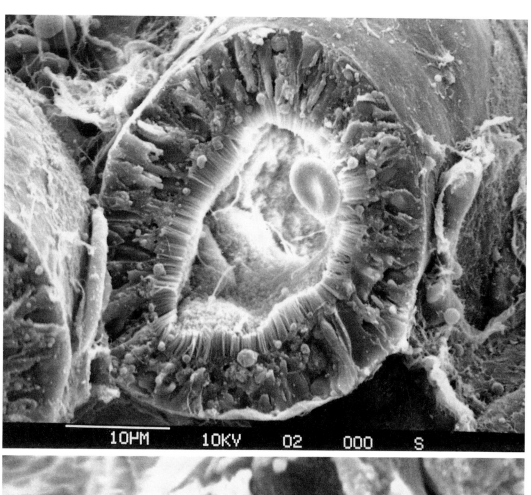

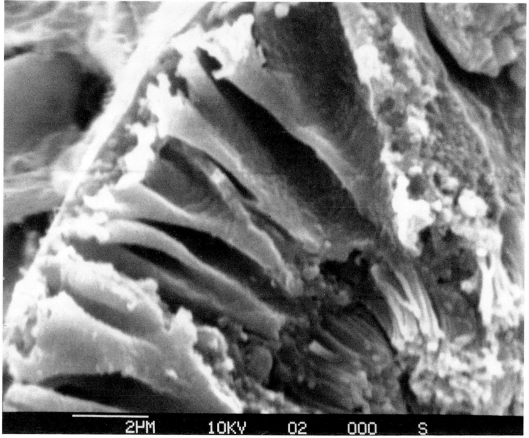

Normal Tubule and Interstitium

Fig. 2-6   Basal infoldings and basal villi of proximal tubule after removal of basement membrane. (scanning electron micrograph, ×10,000)

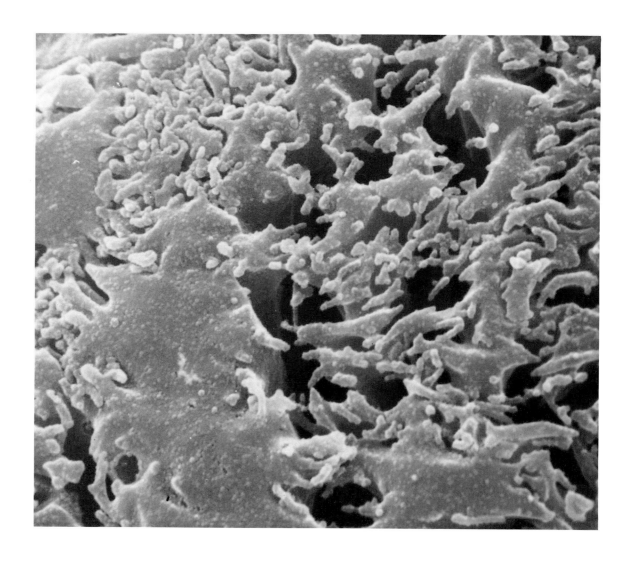

Normal Tubule and Interstitium

Fig. 2-7 Thin segment of loop of Henle, human. (electron micrograph, ×6200)

Fig. 2-8 Distal convoluted tubule, human. Complex, deep invaginations of basal plasmalemma enclose elongated mitochondria. (electron micrograph, ×10,000)

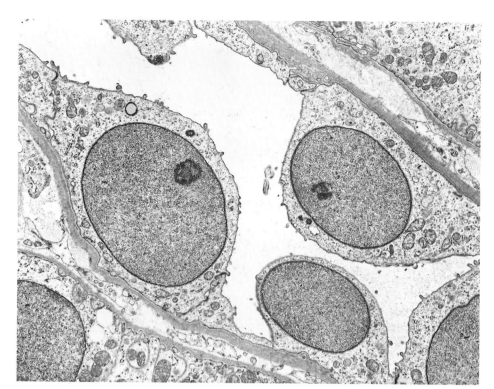

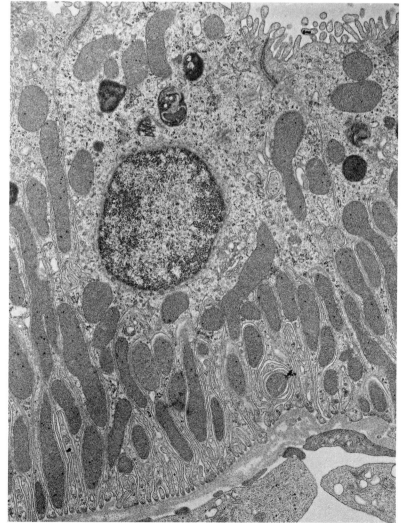

Normal Tubule and Interstitium

Fig. 2-9   Distal convoluted tubule, rabbit. Lateral processes are prominent. (scanning electron micrograph, ×3000)

Fig. 2-10   Cortical collecting duct. Dark cell is in center; parts of light cells are seen on left and right. Dark cell has numerous mitochondria arranged around the nucleus and fairly numerous projections or ridges on the luminal surface. (electron micrograph, ×8400)

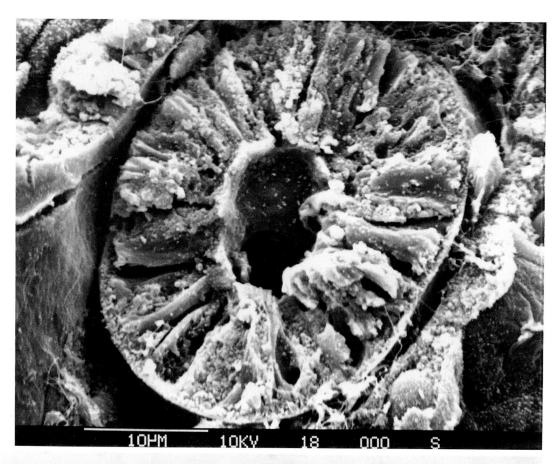

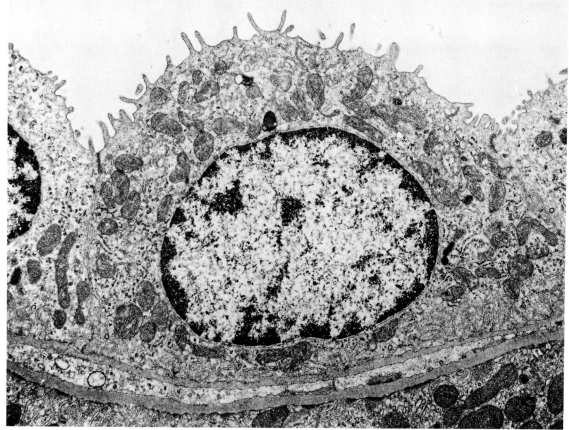

Normal Tubule and Interstitium

Fig. 2-11 Medullary collecting duct, human. Cells are tall and contain only a few organelles. (electron micrograph, ×6300)

Fig. 2-12 Medullary collecting duct, rabbit. Mostly main or light cells are seen. They are equipped with short microvilli and cilia. (scanning electron micrograph, ×5000)

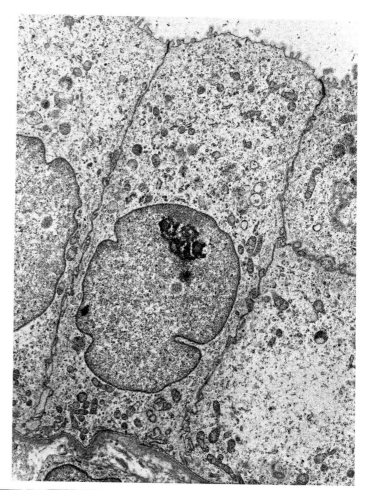

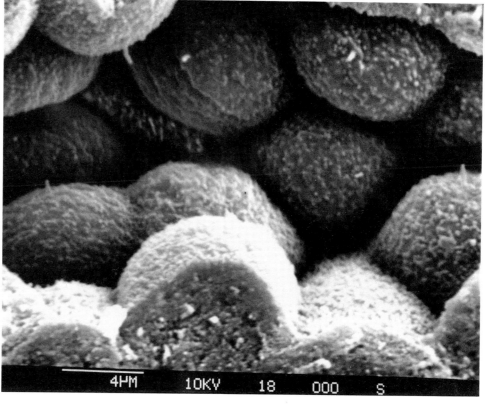

4PM   10KV   18   000   S

Normal Tubule and Interstitium

Fig. 2-13 Interstitial cell (fibroblast) of rabbit kidney showing long cytoplasmic processes, irregularly shaped nucleus and network of fine filaments in peripheral cytoplasm. At one point, the cytoplasm is depressed over the nucleus. Two lipid droplets are present. (electron micrograph, ×16,000)

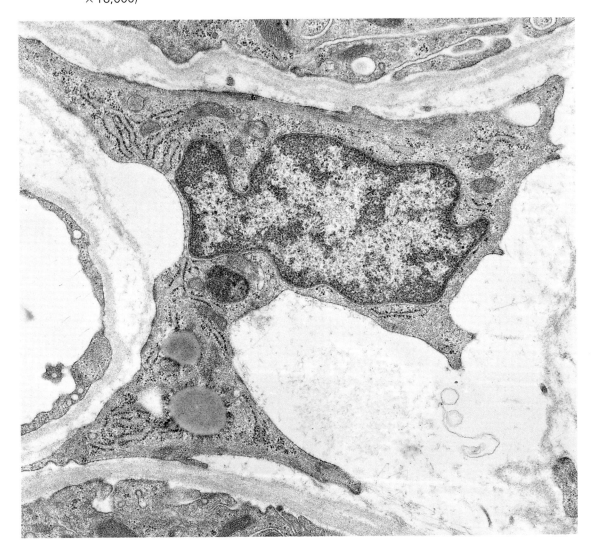

CHAPTER 3

Infection: Acute and Chronic Pyelonephritis

Infection: Acute and Chronic Pyelonephritis

Infection is a major cause of tubulo-interstitial nephritis. In this classification, four different forms of renal involvement are described. The first form is acute infectious tubulo-interstitial nephritis associated with actual proliferation of organisms (bacteria, fungi or viruses) in the renal parenchyma; an example is classical acute bacterial pyelonephritis. The second form is a poorly understood entity in which acute interstitial nephritis is associated with systemic infection but is not caused directly by infectious organisms; clinically, the condition resembles acute drug-induced hypersensitivity tubulo-interstitial nephritis and may well be due to a hypersensitivity reaction. Under the third heading, chronic interstitial nephritis, the most important entity is reflux-associated disease (reflux nephropathy). As will be noted in other sections, although bacteria have an important role in this entity, renal injury may occur in the absence of continued bacterial infection. Last, certain specific infections, such as renal tuberculosis and leprosy, are listed separately.

Acute Infectious Tubulo-interstitial Nephritis (acute pyelonephritis)

Acute Bacterial Tubulo-interstitial Nephritis

This acute inflammatory tubulo-interstitial nephritis is caused by bacterial invasion of the kidneys. It usually is part of a generalized urinary tract infection and ranges in severity from a few scattered foci of inflammation or abscess formation to widespread bilateral suppuration with papillary necrosis. Bacterial invasion of the kidney occurs by ascent from the bladder, most commonly due to vesicoureteral reflux (see Chapter 7), or, less frequently, by hematogenous spread from other foci. By far the most common pathogenic organisms are those of the coliform group, mainly *Escherichia coli,* but many other species can be encountered.

Acute pyelonephritis in male infants occurs with *E. coli* infection predominantly at a ratio of 9:1, and such infants show no anatomic urinary tract abnormality.

Descriptions of the pathologic changes that occur in acute pyelonephritis are based on severely affected kidneys, but studies with laboratory animals have shown that the severity of acute lesions varies considerably; some such lesions affect the pelvic mucosa (pyelitis), whereas other lesions involve entire lobules.

Macroscopic observation indicates that kidneys with severe acute pyelonephritis contain a variable number of abscesses in the cortex and medulla. Occasionally, the areas of inflammation extend from the cortex into the medulla in the shape of a wedge. The papillae may be normal or may show outright papillary necrosis.

Microscopic examination reveals patchy interstitial acute inflammation and tubular necrosis or outright abscess formation. In the presence of ureteral obstruction, the inflammatory reaction sometimes affects an entire kidney.

In experimental acute reflux nephropathy in the pig, large acute inflammatory lesions that correspond to zones of intrarenal reflux have been referred to as "acute lobal nephronia" by Hodson.

Fungal Tubulo-interstitial Nephritis

Fungal infection of the urinary tract is most commonly seen in immunocompromised patients. Fungal infection usually is due to *Candida* species. It may occur secondary to fungemia or may be due to ascending infection. Monilial fungemia usually follows intravenous administration of wide-spectrum antibiotics. It manifests with loin pain and hematuria. Ascending fungal infection usually is due to a foreign body in the bladder (e.g., urinary catheter or stitch). Fungal threads are found in the urine, and such threads may even form fungal balls, which may be seen as space-occupying lesions in the kidney or bladder on excretion urography. Microscopic examination demonstrates fungi and inflammatory reactions in the interstitium, tubules and glomeruli, the latter being an unusual localization for bacterial infection.

Fungi other than *Candida* species rarely infect the urinary tract. *Torulopsis glabrata* can cause cystitis and renal microabscess formation. Other fungi that have been documented as infrequent offending organisms in the causation of urinary tract infection include *Cryptococcus*, *Aspergillus*, *Mucor*, *Histoplasma* and *Blastomyces* species. Involvement of the male genitourinary system is especially common in systemic blastomycosis. *Nocardia* and *Actinomyces* species also have been isolated from infected kidneys, usually secondary to disseminated infection.

Viral Tubulo-interstitial Nephritis

A number of systemic viral illnesses have been associated with viruria, but the role of viruses in renal infection is unclear. Cytomegalovirus infects renal tubules and is a frequent urinary isolate in the cases of systemic infection. Adenovirus type 11 has been recorded as a cause of acute hemorrhagic cystitis, but renal dysfunction is not associated with this syndrome. Adenovirus infection in mice and dogs induces focal interstitial nephritis, but its role in human disease is suspect. A case of severe tubulo-interstitial nephritis associated with BK-type polyomavirus infection has recently been documented. The patient had a hyperglobulin M type of immunodeficiency. The renal disease progressed to irreversible failure.

Acute Tubulo-interstitial Nephritis Associated with Systemic Infection

The term *acute interstitial nephritis* was first used in 1889 by Councilman to describe lesions in the kidneys of patients who died of severe acute infections, particularly scarlet fever and diphtheria, that could not be clearly ascribed to bacterial invasion of the kidneys. The condition was described even earlier as acute lymphomatous nephritis and as a variant of scarlatinal nephritis. Subsequently, other investigators confirmed that the interstitial lesions occurred in the absence of renal invasion by streptococci. This entity has been forgotten because of recent attempts to incriminate a specific drug for every case of acute interstitial nephritis. Yet, a number of well-described cases have been

reported recently in which acute tubulo-interstitial nephritis was associated with bacterial, viral or parasitic infection or with febrile prodromata. Particularly interesting cases have been described with group A streptococcal infections, toxoplasmosis, leptospirosis and Legionnaire's disease. The pathogenesis of these reactions is unknown, but a hypersensitivity reaction is suspected. Histologic examination demonstrates patchy interstitial edema, infiltration with mononuclear cells and tubular degeneration resembling the lesions seen in acute drug-induced hypersensitivity tubulo-interstitial nephritis (see Chapter 6).

Chronic Infectious Tubulo-interstitial Nephritis (chronic pyelonephritis)

Controversy continues to surround the use of the term *chronic pyelonephritis*. Initial confusion arose because of the tendency to equate any chronic tubulo-interstitial damage with bacterial infection, so that most chronic tubulo-interstitial diseases, whatever their etiologic basis, were considered to represent chronic bacterial pyelonephritis. The situation is further clouded by the fact that urinary tract infection is not uncommon in any end-stage chronic renal disease and that bacterial infection of the diseased renal parenchyma may then occur, usually in the terminal stages.

The important distinction to be made is between parenchymal damage resulting from bacterial infection alone ("primary" chronic pyelonephritis) and other forms of tubulo-interstitial disease.

A crucial observation in this respect is that primary infection of the kidneys usually occurs in association with vesicoureteral reflux or urinary tract obstruction resulting from a congenital or acquired urinary tract anomaly. Conversely, urinary tract infection in the absence of obstruction or vesicoureteral reflux rarely causes chronic renal disease.

The morphologic (including the radiologic) features that characterize primary chronic pyelonephritis in association with vesicoureteral reflux are considered below (see also vesicoureteral reflux-associated nephropathy [reflux nephropathy], in Chapter 7). The main criteria are a combination of caliceal deformity with overlying corticomedullary scarring. Only a limited number of other conditions give similar appearances:

1. Analgesic nephropathy (with or without bacterial infection) (see Chapter 5)
2. Unusual forms of noninfectious acute papillary necrosis due to sickle cell disease (see Chapter 8) and dehydration in infants (see Chapter 8)
3. Segmental hypoplasia (Ask-Upmark kidney), a condition now thought to be a type of reflux nephropathy in most instances (see Chapter 7)

Nonobstructive Reflux-Associated Chronic Pyelonephritis

Vesicoureteral Reflux and Intrarenal Reflux

Vesicoureteral reflux describes the return of bladder urine into the ureter during detrusor contraction at micturition due to incompetence of the normal valvular mechanism at the vesicoureteral junction. Vesicoureteral reflux results in the transmission of the increased intravesical pressure during micturition to the renal pelvis. As a result of the rise in intravesical pressure, there is a reversal of the normal pressure gradient between the kidney tubules and the pelvis, so that urine may flow retrogradely from the pelvis into the renal parenchyma (intrarenal reflux). Intrarenal reflux provides a mechanism whereby pathogenic organisms in the bladder urine can gain access to the kidney and initiate scarring. Intrarenal reflux usually occurs only into segments of the kidney that are drained by compound renal papillae. Such segments are located principally at the poles of the kidneys. The smaller conical papillae, which are most prevalent in the midzone of the kidneys, are not normally subject to intrarenal reflux, although their shape may be transformed in the presence of very high pressure vesicoureteral reflux, so that intrarenal reflux and subsequent scarring can then ensue.

Vesicoureteral reflux may result from a primary anomaly of the vesicoureteral junction, or it may be associated with other congenital anomalies of the urinary tract, particularly ureteral ectopia and posterior urethral valve. In such cases, maldifferentiation of the kidneys (renal dysplasia) may occur, and the pathologic changes in the kidneys may represent a combination of those due to congenital maldevelopment and those due to acquired mechanisms. When vesicoureteral reflux occurs, the ureteral orifice is displaced laterally and there is a lack of the normal obliquity of the intramural and submucosal portions of the terminal ureter, on which the competence of the vesicoureteral junction principally depends. Vesicoureteral reflux also may occur as an acquired lesion in patients with neuropathic bladder or dysfunctional voiding and in patients on long-term dialysis.

Reflux Nephropathy

This term describes the corticomedullary scarring that may occur in association with vesicoureteral reflux (see also vesicoureteral reflux-associated nephropathy [reflux nephropathy], in Chapter 7).

Macroscopic Pathology: The characteristic feature of reflux nephropathy is coarse scars, which cause indentation of the renal surface, that lie directly over dilated and deformed ("clubbed") calices. The scars are found to have a wedge shape on section and often are sharply demarcated from adjacent, uninvolved parenchyma, which may undergo compensatory hypertrophy. The site and shape of the scars are readily explained by the mechanism of intrarenal reflux, which initiates their formation. As a result of parenchymal thinning and caliceal dilation, the distance between the calix and the renal capsule may be reduced to a few millimeters in the scars. Usually, not all calices are affected, and scars are most frequent at the poles of the kidneys, where intrarenal reflux occurs most commonly. Occasionally, a single calix is involved, usually at the upper pole. Affected kidneys are smaller than expected, the extent of their diminished size being related to the degree of scarring. Involvement of the kidneys may be unilateral or bilateral; with bilateral involvement, the kidneys often are scarred asymmetrically. When vesicoureteral reflux is associated with mechanical or functional urinary tract obstruction, upper tract dilatation occurs and segmental scarring may be superimposed on varying degrees of diffuse "hydronephrotic" parenchymal atrophy of the kidney (see Chapter 7).

Microscopic Findings: Within scarred areas, the changes are predominantly tubulo-interstitial, and appearances vary according to the stage of evolution of the lesion. Old scars may be composed almost entirely of atrophic tubules, which often are dilated and filled with eosinophilic casts (so-called thyroidization), separated by fibrous tissue. More recent scars usually exhibit interstitial chronic inflammation, often with prominent lymphoid follicle formation. When this change is associated with similar chronic inflammatory changes of the renal pelvis and ureter, it is an indication of active renal infection. Tubular casts that contain polymorphonuclear neutrophils also may be observed under these conditions. Glomerular changes (periglomerular fibrosis, ischemic atrophy and global sclerosis) are observed when scarring is advanced; the glomeruli often appear crowded together as a result of loss of intervening tissue. Arteriosclerosis (fibroelastic intimal thickening of arteries and hyaline thickening of arteriolar walls) may be a feature in the scars, even in the absence of hypertension. When this complication occurs, vascular changes tend to be more generalized and may affect arteries and arterioles in scarred and unscarred areas of the parenchyma. Occasionally, foci of dysplastic elements may be seen.

A glomerular lesion, which resembles focal glomerulosclerosis and hyalinosis on the basis of histologic criteria, that affects unscarred areas of the kidneys has recently been described in patients with reflux nephropathy, and usually is associated clinically with proteinuria and a tendency toward progressive renal failure (see Classification and Atlas of Glomerular Diseases).

Radiologic Features: At excretion urography, the scarred kidney of reflux nephropathy is found to be variably smaller and to show areas of parenchymal thinning ("scarring") relating to deformed ("clubbed") calices, most frequently at the poles of the kidney. There may or may not be upper tract dilatation. Involvement may be unilateral or bilateral; with bilateral involvement, the extent of the changes often differs between the two sides. Vesicoureteral reflux can be demonstrated on micturating cystourethrography in about 0.5% of unselected children, but its frequency is influenced by genetic variables because several recent studies have shown an incidence of between 8% and 26% in siblings of patients known to have the lesion. Conversely, between 30% and 60% of all children with vesicoureteral reflux have renal scarring. The "severity" of the lesion is determined conventionally on a grading system, with higher grades exhibiting upper tract dilatation; there is a tendency for renal scarring to be more frequent and more severe with the higher grades of reflux (see Chapter 7). Vesicoureteral reflux tends to remit spontaneously with time in most children, so that older children and adults with reflux nephropathy often fail to demonstrate reflux on radiologic examination. Spontaneous remission of reflux is much commoner with low-grade reflux.

Patients with segmental renal scarring associated with vesicoureteral reflux usually have scars when first seen by a physician (before five years of age), and the development of new scars in a previously normal kidney is uncommon after that age. This observation strongly suggests that scarring occurs during early childhood and probably during infancy.

Other Variants

Chronic nonobstructive pyelonephritis in the absence of vesicoureteral reflux is at best an ill-defined entity. Vesicoureteral reflux often remits spontaneously, so that associated renal scarring occasionally is discovered only when reflux can no longer be demonstrated. Some patients with urinary tract infection may be judged on the basis of clinical criteria to have renal infection without vesicoureteral reflux or urinary tract obstruction. Pathologic verification of renal involvement is necessarily lacking, but the radiologic evidence does not suggest that serious renal scarring has occurred.

Chronic Obstructive Pyelonephritis

Associated with Urinary Tract Obstruction

The effects of urinary tract obstruction are defined and described in Chapter 7. Urinary tract obstruction predisposes to an increased incidence of urinary tract infection, acute or chronic.

Pathology: Macroscopic Findings: In chronic obstructive pyelonephritis, where mechanical obstruction can be demonstrated in the ureter or lower urinary tract, the pathologic (and radiologic) changes are a combination of those due to obstruc-

tion and those due to infection. The renal pelvis and calices are dilated, and the thickness of the renal parenchyma is uniformly reduced. In pure obstructive uropathy uncomplicated by infection, the subcapsular surface of the kidney usually is surprisingly smooth, whereas when infection is present, it often is granular. Occasionally, particularly when obstruction is due to renal calculi, the changes seen in xanthogranulomatous pyelonephritis (see Chapter 4) may be encountered.

In some cases, areas of segmental scarring, similar to those seen in reflux nephropathy, may be superimposed. Experimental observations in pigs with acute obstruction in association with infection indicate that such segmental scarring may result from intrarenal reflux of infected urine; the reflux in this setting is a result of increased intrapelvic pressure, which is due to vigorous pelvic and ureteral peristalsis sufficient to reverse the pressure gradient between the pelvis and the renal parenchyma. It is probable that a similar mechanism may explain the segmental scarring seen in chronic obstructive pyelonephritis in human beings.

It should be recognized, too, that an obstructive agent is present in many cases of reflux nephropathy. In some settings, such as posterior urethral valve, urinary tract obstruction and vesicoureteral reflux coexist. In addition, when vesicoureteral reflux is associated with marked ureteral dilatation, the column of urine in the expanded upper tract itself constitutes a functional obstructive element. In either event, diffuse pelvicaliceal dilatation and parenchymal atrophy as well as segmental scarring associated with intrarenal reflux may ensue.

Microscopic Findings: In addition to changes attributable to obstruction alone (see pathologic changes in the kidneys, in Chapter 7), active parenchymal infection is associated with focal or diffuse chronic interstitial inflammation, usually with prominent lymphoid follicle formation. Chronic inflammation of the pelvicaliceal system and ureter also are indications of infection.

Acute Bacterial Tubulo-interstitial Nephritis (acute pyelonephritis)

Fig. 3-1   Kidney showing numerous cortical abscesses.

Fig. 3-2   Small cortical abscesses on cut surface of another kidney.

Fig. 3-3   Cortical abscess. Histologic section from the same case as in Figure 3-2. (hematoxylin and eosin, ×110)

Fig. 3-4   Bacterial colony in center of abscess. (hematoxylin and eosin, ×430)

Fig. 3-5   Large cortical abscess (carbuncle) extending into the medulla (left side of picture).

Fig. 3-6   Low magnification of streaks of pus in medulla. (hematoxylin and eosin, ×30)

Fig. 3-7   Higher magnification of Figure 3-6 showing pus casts in tubular lumina. (hematoxylin and eosin, ×200)

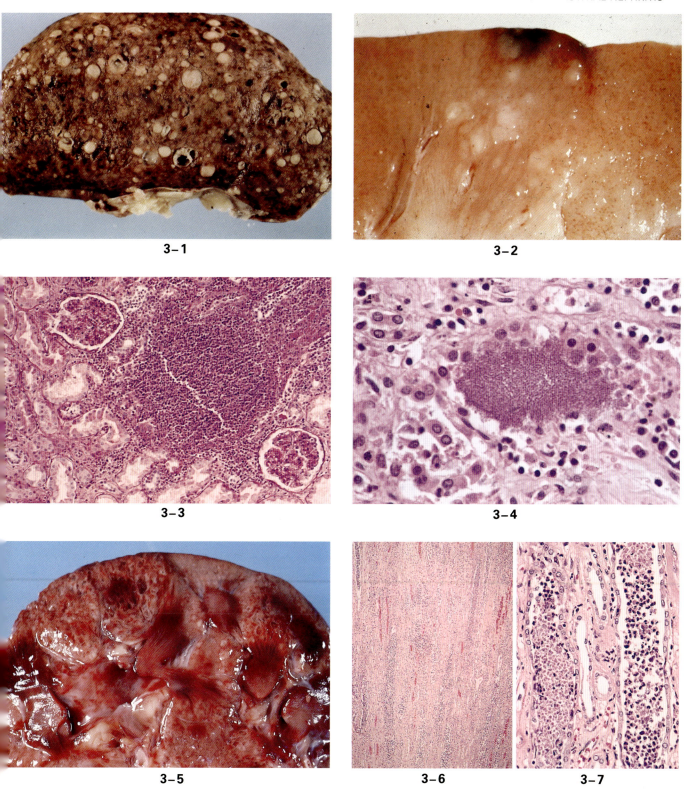

3–1

3–2

3–3

3–4

3–5

3–6

3–7

Fungal Tubulo-interstitial Nephritis

Fig. 3-8   Histoplasmosis. Cut surface showing small white cortical nodules in immunocompromised patient (treated lymphoma).

Fig. 3-9   Histoplasmosis. Same case as in Figure 3-8. Histologic section of one nodule showing chronic granulomatous inflammation. (hematoxylin and eosin, ×70)

Fig. 3-10 Histoplasmosis. *Histoplasma capsulatum* in a granulomatous nodule. (Gram-methenamine silver, ×430)

Fig. 3-11 Mucormycosis. Hyphae surrounded by macrophages. (Grocott's silver, ×270)

Fig. 3-12 *Candida albicans (Monilia)*. Abscess containing yeastlike organisms and hyphae. (periodic acid-Schiff, ×430)

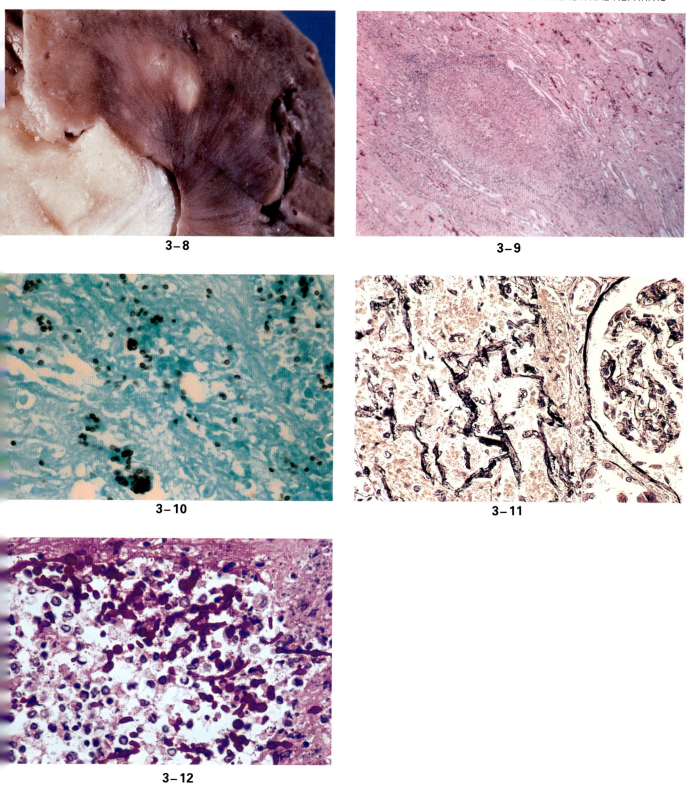

3-8

3-9

3-10

3-11

3-12

Viral Tubulo-interstitial Nephritis

Fig. 3-13 Cytomegalovirus infection. Viral inclusions in tubular epithelial cells accompanied by interstitial inflammation in child with immunodeficiency syndrome. (hematoxylin and eosin, ×270)

Fig. 3-14 Cytomegalovirus infection. Higher magnification of infected tubular cells. (hematoxylin and eosin, ×550)

Chronic Infectious Tubulo-interstitial Nephritis (chronic pyelonephritis)

Fig. 3-15 Chronic pyelonephritis. Numerous deep cortical scars.

Fig. 3-16 Chronic nonobstructive pyelonephritis. Numerous cortical scars, more prominent at poles.

Fig. 3-17 Chronic pyelonephritis. Marked narrowing of parenchyma, dilatation of calix and chronic submucosal inflammation. (hematoxylin and eosin, ×10)

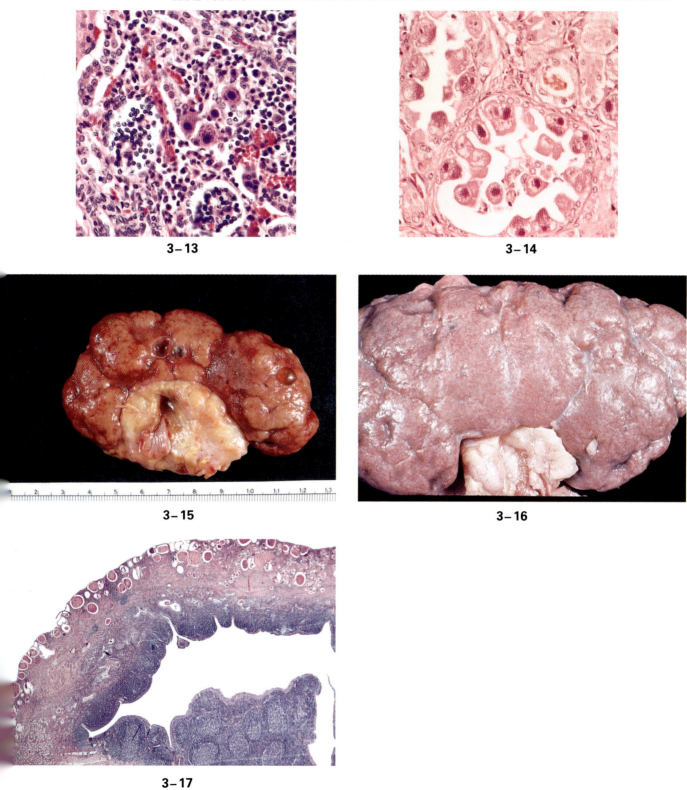

3-13

3-14

3-15

3-16

3-17

Chronic Infectious Tubulo-interstitial Nephritis (chronic pyelonephritis)

Fig. 3-18 Severe interstitial inflammation with destruction of tubules and peri-glomerular fibrosis. (hematoxylin and eosin, × 110)

Fig. 3-19 Chronic interstitial inflammation and fibrosis, sclerosis of glomeruli and arteriosclerosis. (trichrome, × 70)

Fig. 3-20 Chronic interstitial inflammation and many dilated tubules filled with hyaline casts (''thyroidization''). (hematoxylin and eosin, × 110)

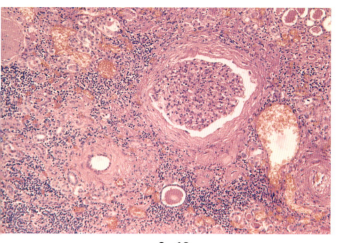

3–18

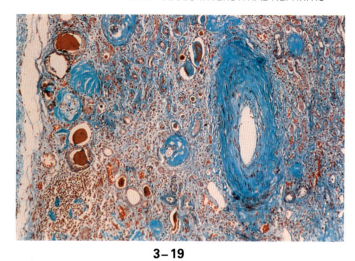

3–19

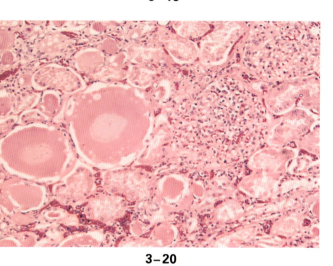

3–20

CHAPTER 4

Infection: Special Forms of Pyelonephritis

Infection: Special Forms of Pyelonephritis

Xanthogranulomatous Pyelonephritis

This type of chronic bacterial tubulo-interstitial nephritis is characterized by granulomas, abscesses, collections of lipid-filled macrophages (foam cells) and severe renal parenchymal destruction.

Clinical Features: The disease is almost always unilateral. Most patients have a history of calculus disease, obstructive uropathy or diabetes mellitus; a renal mass is present in 60% of cases.

Macroscopic Findings: The affected kidney is enlarged, and the capsule and perirenal tissue are thickened and adherent. The process may be localized to one tumor mass or may be diffuse and multifocal. The renal parenchyma, particularly that which surrounds the dilated calices, is replaced by orange-yellow, soft inflammatory tissue, often with small abscesses. The renal mass can be mistaken grossly for renal cell carcinoma, but the coexistence of stones, obstruction and abscesses and the localization of yellow tissue near the calices suggest an inflammatory disorder.

Microscopic Findings: The inflammatory tissue consists of an admixture of large foamy macrophages, smaller macrophages with granular cyto-plasm, neutrophils, lymphocytes, plasma cells, fibroblasts and occasional histiocytic giant cells. The cytoplasm of the foamy macrophages and the small granular monocytes stain strongly with periodic acid-Schiff. *Intravenous pyelography* frequently demonstrates caliceal deformities and irregularities, in the diffuse type. Localized lesions appear as cystic masses. Angiography reveals that most xanthogranulomatous renal masses are hypovascular or avascular. Urine cultures are almost invariably positive. *Proteus mirabilis* is cultured most frequently, although in some series, *E. coli* has been found more often.

The pathogenesis of xanthogranulomatous pyelonephritis is unclear, although it seems certain that the condition is caused by bacterial infection accentuated by urinary tract obstruction. Electron microscopy shows that the macrophages initially contain bacteria; subsequently, phagolysosomes filled with myelin figures and amorphous material are observed, suggesting a lysosomal defect that interferes with the digestion of bacterial products.

Malacoplakia

This condition, usually confined to the urinary bladder, also affects the kidneys and other organs.

It is most common in middle-aged women who have chronic urinary tract infection and in immunosuppressed patients. The microscopic lesions are typical, being composed of large, closely packed macrophages with occasional lymphocytes and multinucleated giant cells. The macrophages have abundant, foamy, periodic acid-Schiff-positive cytoplasm. In addition, laminated, mineralized concretions, known as Michaelis-Gutmann bodies, are typically present within macrophages and in the interstitial tissue. Electron microscopy demonstrates that these bodies have a typical crystalline structure with a dense central core, an intermediate halo and a lamellated peripheral ring.

Renal malacoplakia occurs in the same clinical setting as xanthogranulomatous pyelonephritis, namely, chronic infection and obstruction. *E. coli* is the most common organism that is cultured from the urine. Bilateral involvement has been reported, as has a clinical presentation that simulates acute renal failure.

Megalocytic Interstitial Nephritis

This condition is characterized by nodular or diffuse infiltration of the renal interstitium by large polygonal macrophages, similar to those seen in malacoplakia. The gross appearance of an affected kidney also may be similar. In some cases, which probably represent a minor variant of malacoplakia, the macrophages stain intensely with periodic acid-Schiff. However, in other cases, the macrophages do not stain, and additional features, such as small necrotizing granulomas, may be encountered. Electron-lucent, crystalloid structures in the macrophagic phagolysosomes also have been reported.

Specific Renal Infections

A variety of infectious agents can induce various forms of tubulo-interstitial disease. Variants of the disease induced by infectious agents include tuberculosis, leprosy, epidemic hemorrhagic fever (e.g., dengue) and many other bacterial and parasitic infections.

Tuberculosis

Renal tuberculosis results from the hematogenous spread of mycobacteria from the lungs and usually is discovered when there is active lung disease. Clinical features of renal tuberculosis include dysuria and hematuria, with fever and loss of weight. There may be coincidental tuberculous cystitis, prostatitis, ureteritis, epididymitis or salpingitis.

Macroscopic Findings: In miliary tuberculosis, there are many small white cortical nodules. In tuberculous pyonephrosis, the renal parenchyma is involved by large, confluent, white, soft, cheesy necrotic masses. Early lesions are found in the medulla and papillae, with later involvement of the pelvis and cortex with thick, cheesy material. Secondary hydronephrosis may occur with ureteral obstruction and strictures.

Microscopic Findings: Typical features of tuberculous granulomatous reaction include macrophages and leukocytes, mainly epithelioid cells and lymphocytes, with varying numbers of Langhans'-type multinucleated giant cells. There is caseous necrosis, and acid- and alcohol-fast bacilli should be identified with Ziehl-Neelsen's stain. Older lesions may show calcification. Surrounding renal parenchyma shows tubulo-interstitial fibrosis and lymphocytic infiltrates, with periglomerular fibrosis.

Leprosy

In this chronic infectious disease caused by *Mycobacterium leprae*, the type of lesion (lepromatous leprosy, tuberculoid variety or borderline forms) depends on the host's immune response.

Three different types of renal involvement have been described:

1. Glomerular lesions suggestive of circulating immune complex glomerulonephritis with granular deposits of IgG, C3 and, to a lesser extent, IgM. The glomeruli show variable morphologic features, with diffuse mesangial cell proliferation, endocapillary proliferation, focal proliferation and mesangial sclerosis.
2. Renal amyloidosis occurs in 5% to 30% of cases reported from Africa, India and the United States. It is more frequent in the lepromatous form of leprosy, and the changes are the same as in any form of secondary amyloidosis.
3. Tubulo-interstitial involvement is not a major lesion in leprosy. The impairment of renal tubular function in the absence of tubulo-interstitial lesions has been attributed to immunologic abnormalities.

Syphilis

Renal involvement in syphilis is now rare, but such involvement may be seen in congenital syphilis and in the secondary and tertiary stages of acquired disease. There may be immune complex glomerulonephritis with deposits of IgG and C3 in the mesangium and capillary loops, together with proliferative and membranous lesions.

Interstitial nephritis is now rare, but in the past its incidence had been reported to be as high as 6.5% of adult cases of confirmed syphilis. Some degree of albuminuria is found, but nephrotic syndrome is unusual and renal failure is uncommon.

Macroscopic Findings: Small gray patches are seen on the subcapsular surface, which on section are found to extend down into the medulla.

Microscopic Findings: Focal mononuclear infiltrates, predominantly plasma cells, are seen in the interstitium and around blood vessels. There also is evidence of interstitial edema. The proximal convoluted tubules show varying degrees of degeneration, with swelling and necrosis of epithelial cells and zones of dilated tubules containing eosinophilic casts. In advanced stages, there is tubular atrophy and interstitial fibrosis. Immunofluorescence may demonstrate deposition of IgG around the tubules and in the interstitium.

Epidemic Hemorrhagic Fever

Outbreaks of hemorrhagic fever appear periodically around the world. Dengue hemorrhagic fever, an arboviral disease transmitted by the tiger mosquito, *Aedes aegypti*, occurs on the Asian mainland as an endemic infectious disease. Epidemic hemorrhagic fever with acute tubulo-interstitial nephritis occurs predominantly in northern Scandinavia and Finland as nephritis epidemica. Clinical studies have shown that a number of patients have a mild form of epidemic hemorrhagic fever. Shock may occur at any stage, and patients with severe renal failure may have had slight transient or no preceding hypotension. The onset is abrupt, with fever, headache and malaise.

Abdominal or loin pain develops after four to five days, often with severe proteinuria. Slight oliguria and azotemia also are common, and the oliguria may progress to acute anuria of short duration. Recovery with polyuria usually begins after eight to 10 days and is complete after two or three weeks. No persistent abnormality of renal function has been described. The clinical picture in nephritis epidemica is similar to those of dengue hemorrhagic fever and hemorrhagic fever with renal syndrome (seen in the Soviet Union), but the prognosis is much better in patients with nephritis epidemica. Generalized hemorrhagic symptoms are uncommon in nephritis epidemica, which is caused by a virus that is closely related but not identical to the virus that causes dengue hemorrhagic fever. The vector animals for both viruses are rodents (mice, rats and voles).

Macroscopic Findings: At autopsy, the kidneys are found to be enlarged, the cortex is pale and the medulla is congested. Submucosal hemorrhages and petechiae often are seen in the renal pelvis.

Microscopic Findings: The glomerular changes are mild or minimal and include occasional segmental adhesions between capillaries and Bowman's capsule. The main changes are interstitial edema and hemorrhage in the cortex and medulla.

There are focal lymphocytic infiltrates in the interstitium. Red blood cells may be present in the tubular lumina. The tubular epithelial cells may show degeneration and necrosis; focal areas of anoxic tubular necrosis with cytoplasmic hyaline droplets occur in proximal tubules, and flattened degenerating cells are seen in the distal tubules. Mild tubular atrophy and peritubular fibrosis may persist for many years without impairment of renal function. The cause of the oliguria or anuria may be increased intrarenal pressure due to interstitial edema in combination with hemorrhage and shock. There is no evidence of obstruction of nephrons by red cell casts.

Other: Tropical infections and parasitic infestations of the kidney will be discussed in the volume on Infectious and Tropical Diseases of the Kidney.

Xanthogranulomatous Pyelonephritis

Fig. 4-1 Xanthogranulomatous pyelonephritis. Localized lesion simulating tumor.

Fig. 4-2 Extensive lesions showing yellow periphery and congested hemorrhagic centers.

Fig. 4-3 Almost complete replacement of kidney by yellow hemorrhagic masses and fibrous tissue.

Fig. 4-4 Numerous foamy histiocytes and chronic inflammatory cells in renal interstitium. (hematoxylin and eosin, ×160)

Fig. 4-5 Higher magnification of Figure 4-4 showing foamy histiocytes and numerous plasma cells. (hematoxylin and eosin, ×430)

Fig. 4-6 Many broken down foamy cells and cholesterol crystal clefts. (hematoxylin and eosin, ×160)

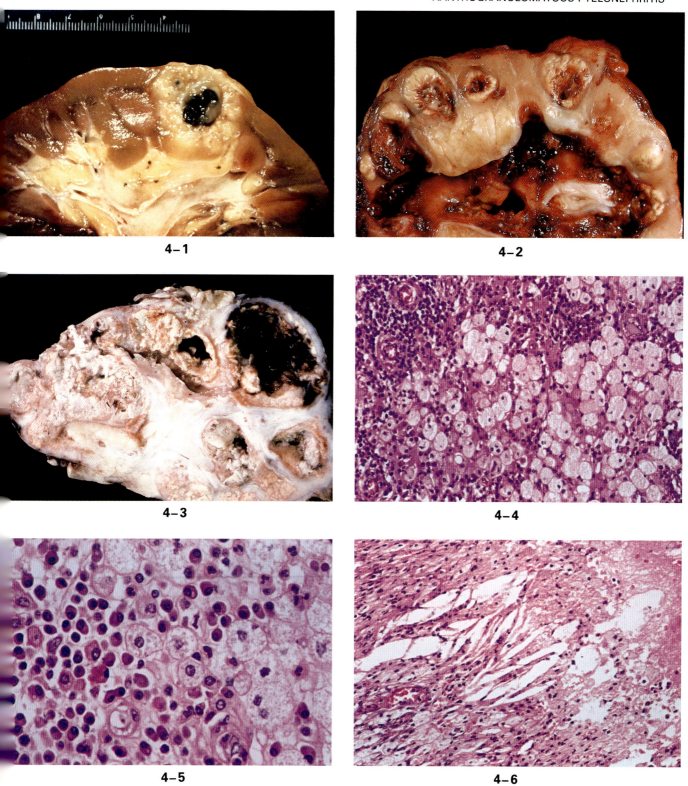

4–1

4–2

4–3

4–4

4–5

4–6

Malacoplakia

Fig. 4-7   Malacoplakia. Numerous yellow nodules on surface of kidney.

Fig. 4-8   Advanced stage of malacoplakia with extensive replacement of parenchyma.

Fig. 4-9   Cut surface of advanced stage showing almost complete replacement of cortex. Medullary markings are still noticeable. (fixed specimen)

Fig. 4-10 Massive accumulation of large histiocytes with vesicular nuclei and pale cytoplasm. Scattered inflammatory cells also are present. (hematoxylin and eosin, ×430)

Fig. 4-11 Histiocytes filled with periodic acid-Schiff-positive material. (periodic acid-Schiff, ×430)

Fig. 4-12 Numerous Michaelis-Gutmann bodies. (von Kossa's stain, ×430)

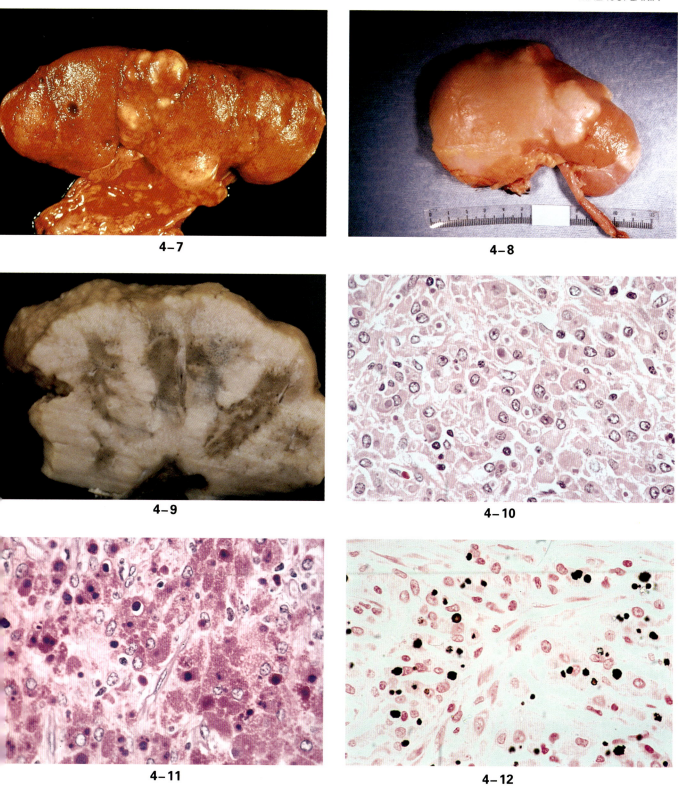

4-7

4-8

4-9

4-10

4-11

4-12

Megalocytic Interstitial Nephritis

Fig. 4-13 Megalocytic interstitial nephritis. Extensive replacement of renal paren-chyma by densely packed histiocytes. (hematoxylin and eosin, ×110)

Fig. 4-14 In this disease, histiocytes do not stain with periodic acid-Schiff, whereas they do stain in malacoplakia. (periodic acid-Schiff, ×430)

Fig. 4-15 Same case as in Figure 4-14. Another area of kidney showing chronic granulomatous inflammation with central necrosis. (hematoxylin and eosin, ×270)

Fig. 4-16 Second biopsy specimen from the same case as in Figures 4-14 and 4-15, 10 years later. During this period, the patient had repeated attacks of interstitial nephritis with renal insufficiency, which responded par-tially to Corticosteroid therapy. At this time, the patient is in renal failure. There is extensive tubular atrophy and focal chronic inflammation. His-tiocytes seen in the previous biopsy specimen have disappeared. Glo-meruli show various degrees of sclerosis. (periodic acid-Schiff, ×110)

Fig. 4-17 Same case as in Figure 4-16. Tubular atrophy with vacuolation of tubular cells. (hematoxylin and eosin, ×270)

Fig. 4-18 Same case as in Figure 4-17. Interstitial fibrosis and chronic inflam-mation, tubular atrophy and tubular cell hyperplasia. (hematoxylin and eosin, ×110)

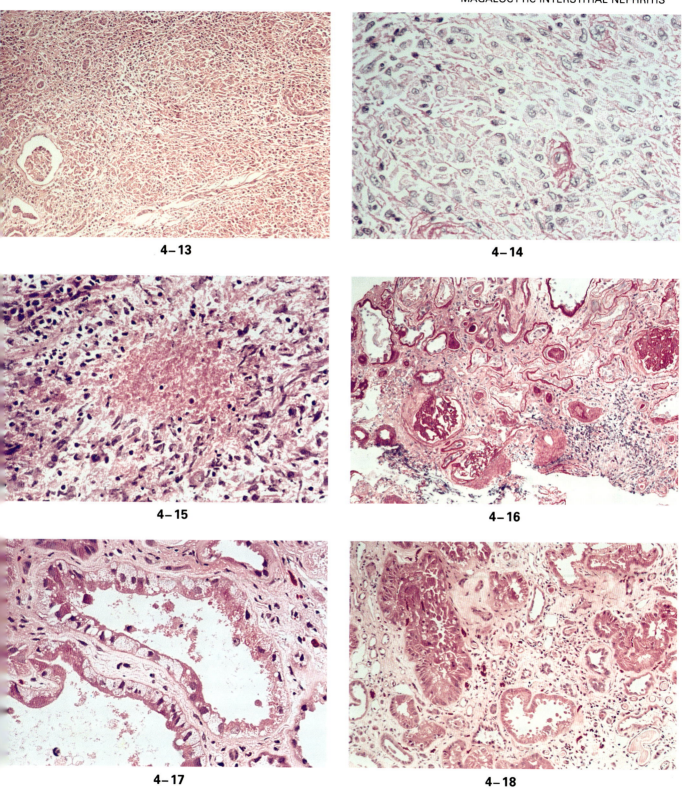

4–13

4–14

4–15

4–16

4–17

4–18

Specific Renal Infections
Tuberculosis

Fig. 4-19 Miliary tuberculosis. Numerous yellowish-white nodules on surface of kidney.

Fig. 4-20 Miliary tuberculosis. Caseating granuloma centered on a glomerulus. (periodic acid-Schiff, ×270)

Fig. 4-21 Ulcerating, caseating tuberculosis of kidney extending into ureters and bladder.

Fig. 4-22 Contracted, fibrocaseous tuberculosis with involvement of ureter.

Fig. 4-23 Tuberculous granulomata in cortex of kidney. (hematoxylin and eosin, ×160)

Fig. 4-24 Caseating tuberculous granuloma. (hematoxylin and eosin, ×270)

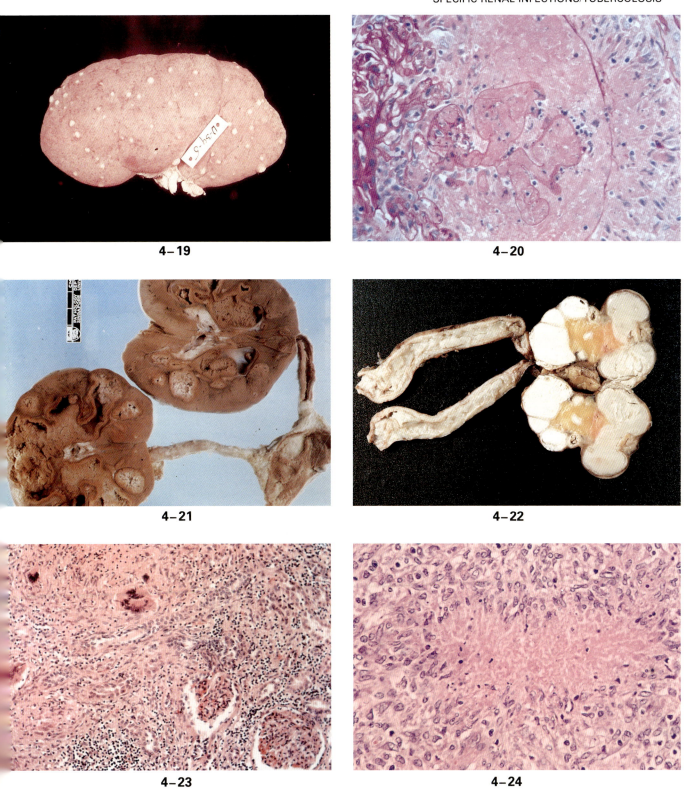

4-19

4-20

4-21

4-22

4-23

4-24

Leprosy

Fig. 4-25 Leprosy. Granulomatous tubulo-interstitial inflammation. (hematoxylin and eosin, ×150)

Fig. 4-26 Leprosy. Acid-fast bacilli in "lepra" cells. (Fites stain, ×540)

Syphilis

Fig. 4-27 Syphilis. Chronic interstitial inflammation, tubular atrophy and fibrosis and arterial intimal thickening. (hematoxylin and eosin, ×80)

Epidemic Hemorrhagic Fever (nephritis epidemica)

Fig. 4-28 Epidemic hemorrhagic fever. Marked congestion of kidney and beginning of tubular necrosis. (hematoxylin and eosin, ×135)

Fig. 4-29 Nephritis epidemica. Extensive tubular necrosis and interstitial inflammation. (hematoxylin and eosin, ×135)

Fig. 4-30 Same case as in Figure 4-29. Interstitial edema and inflammation at corticomedullary junction. (hematoxylin and eosin, ×135)

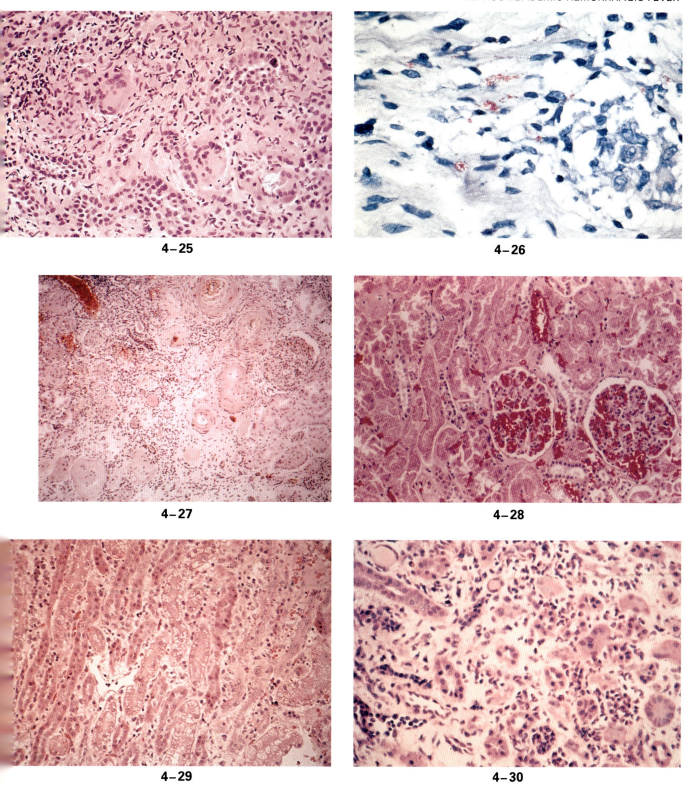

4–25

4–26

4–27

4–28

4–29

4–30

Xanthogranulomatous Pyelonephritis

Fig. 4-31 Xanthogranulomatous pyelonephritis. Typical "foamy" macrophages and disintegrating cells containing bacteria. (electron micrograph, ×6600)

Fig. 4-32 Xanthogranulomatous pyelonephritis. Bacteria in cell cytoplasm. (electron micrograph, ×22,000)

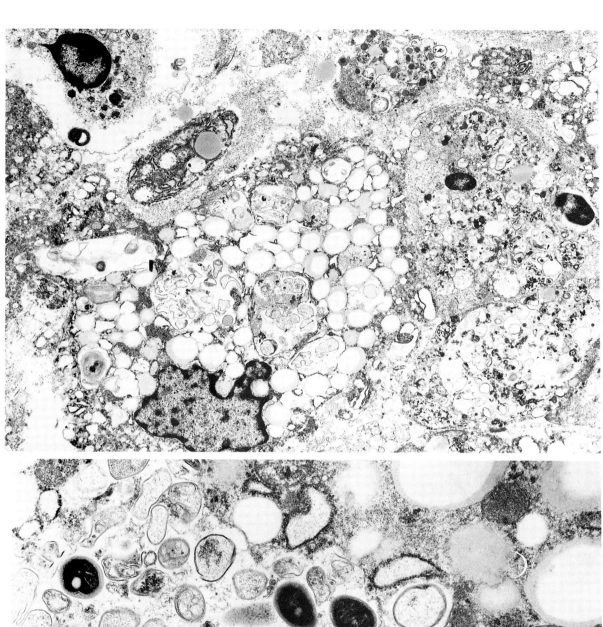
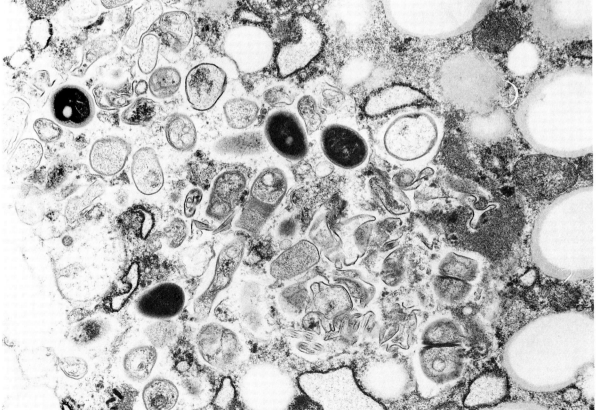

Xanthogranulomatous Pyelonephritis

Fig. 4-33 Xanthogranulomatous pyelonephritis. X-ray appearance of large mass in upper renal pole consisting of central abscess surrounded by fibrosis, inflammation and xanthogranulomatous nodules. Staghorn calculus also is visible.

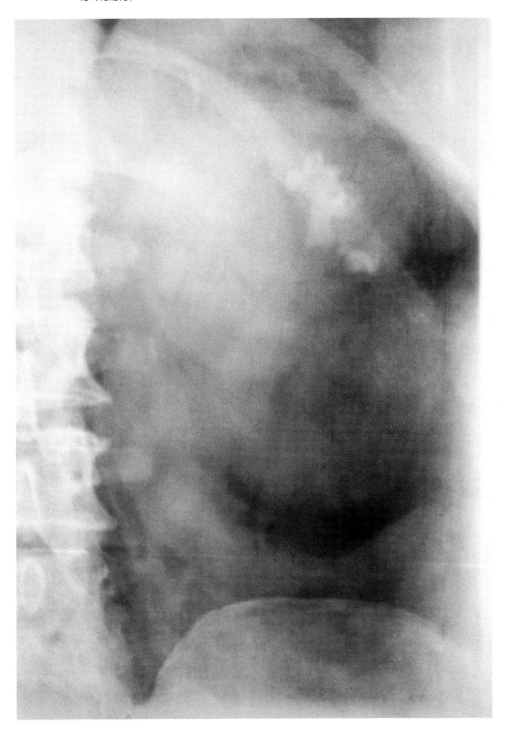

Xanthogranulomatous Pyelonephritis

Fig. 4-34 Same case as in Figure 4-33. Urogram showing pressure distortion of caliceal system by renal mass.

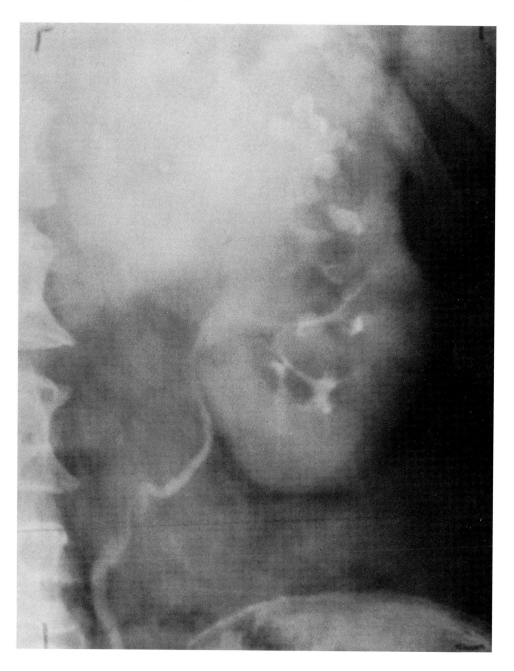

Xanthogranulomatous Pyelonephritis

Fig. 4-35 Same case as in Figure 4-34. Selective left renal angiogram showing abnormal vessels in mass, especially at periphery, with displacement of capsular vessels away from surface of kidney.

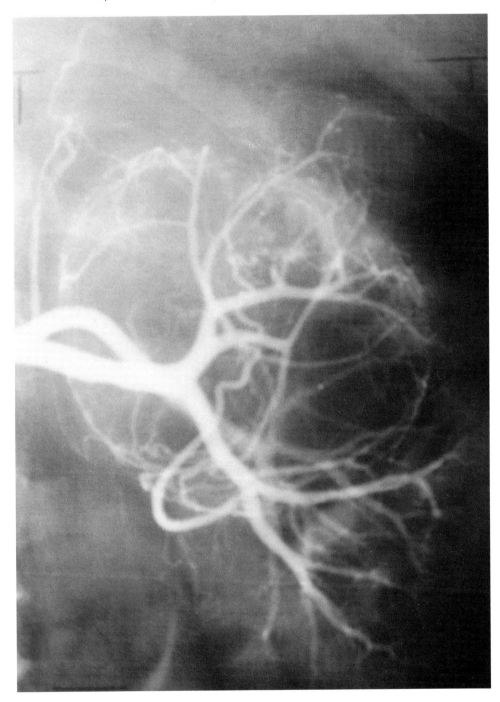

Malacoplakia

Fig. 4-36 Malacoplakia. Bacteria (probably *Escherichia coli*) in disrupted macrophage. (electron micrograph, ×16,000)

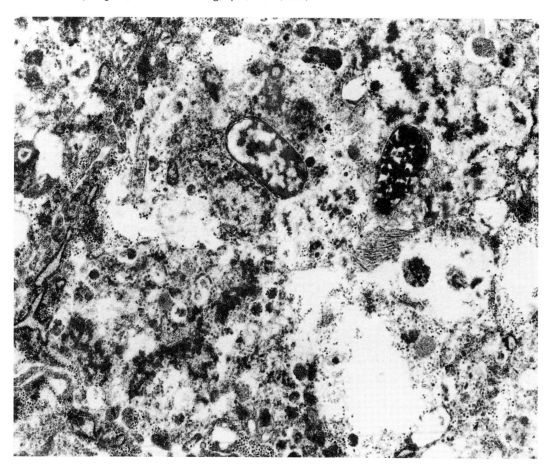

Malacoplakia

Fig. 4-37 Malacoplakia. Well-developed, concentric Michaelis-Gutmann body. (electron micrograph, ×4000)

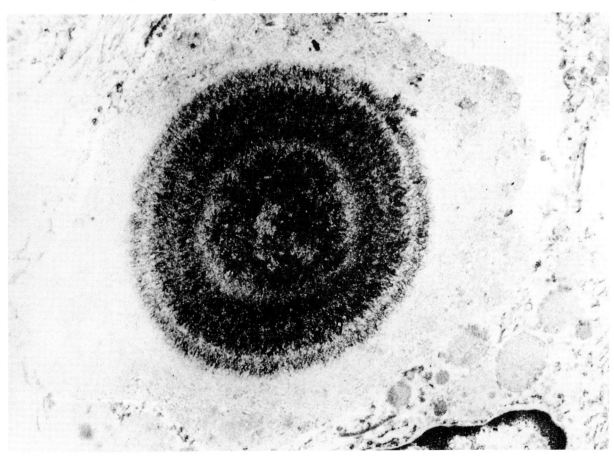

CHAPTER 5

Drug-Induced Tubulo-interstitial Nephritis

Drug-Induced Tubulo-interstitial Nephritis

Drug-induced tubulo-interstitial nephritis is an acute disease related to ingestion of a normal or large dose of a drug. The disease affects mainly the tubular system and the renal interstitium. However, in some cases, the disease may be recurrent or chronic.

The acute form of the disease usually is caused by acute tubulotoxic injury or by a hypersensitivity reaction either (a) directly or (b) indirectly from effects on other systems (e.g. hemolysis from chloroquine or hypokalemia). Tetracyclines may cause natriuresis and tubular necrosis with renal failure. Tubulotoxicity is a direct result of damage induced by the offending drug and in most cases is a dose-related phenomenon, whereas allergic reactions are assumed to be due to immunologic processes that are elicited by the drug when it functions as a hapten, and circulating or structural proteins. Such reactions are not dose-related occurrences. The exact mechanism may not be known, or the two pathways may be combined.

There must be a causal and/or temporal relationship between drug intake and onset of clinical symptoms. However, because the latent period from drug ingestion to onset of symptoms is variable, ranging from a few hours to more than one week, and because some offending drugs (e.g., antibiotics) are taken at frequent intervals, such a relationship often is difficult to establish.

Acute Tubulotoxic Injury (see acute tubular necrosis, Chapter 10)

Drug-Induced Hypersensitivity Tubulo-interstitial Nephritis

This form of tubulo-interstitial nephritis is characterized by fever, nausea, vomiting, acute renal insufficiency, microscopic or macroscopic hematuria and an accelerated erythrocyte sedimentation rate. Skin exanthema and blood eosinophilia sometimes occur. Nevertheless, the full clinical picture is not always present. In most cases, clinical resolution occurs soon after ingestion of the offending drug has been discontinued. Corticosteroids have been reported to produce a beneficial effect. Chronic renal insufficiency rarely occurs.

Macroscopic Findings: Both kidneys are enlarged, pale or reddened and soft. On sectioning, the corticomedullary junction often is found to be indistinct.

Microscopic Findings: The histologic picture is not specific and includes interstitial edema and cellular infiltrates composed mainly of lymphocytes and plasma cells without marked fibrosis. The infiltrates are patchy or, in severe cases, diffuse.

Eosinophilic granulocytes are found in about 25% of cases. Granulomas may be seen, especially in methicillin- or sulfonamide-induced tubulo-interstitial nephritis. Tubular epithelial cells may be swollen or flattened and sometimes are exfoliated or necrosed. Severe tubular destruction is rare, but "tubulorrhexic" lesions are not an uncommon occurrence (see p. 138).

Although the glomeruli are mostly unaltered, they may show a low-grade increase in mesangial cells. In most cases, pathologic alterations are not found in vessels, although vasculitis has been described. Immunofluorescence studies may demonstrate granular deposits of immunoglobulins and/or complement in the interstitium as well as in the glomeruli or vessels, but such studies usually reveal no abnormality, especially if the biopsy is done more than six to eight weeks after the onset of the disease. Linear deposition of immunoglobulins along tubular basement membranes is rare.

Chronic Drug-Induced Tubulo-interstitial Nephritis

Analgesic Nephropathy

A chronic tubulo-interstitial kidney disease, analgesic nephropathy is caused by heavy usage of analgesic compounds that contain phenacetin and/or aspirin (acetylsalicylic acid). The prevalence of the disease appears to vary among different geographic areas.

Clinical Features: Renal papillary necrosis in association with a history of long-term analgesic abuse is indicative of analgesic nephropathy. The finding of necrotic tissue in the urine is evidence of papillary necrosis; more commonly, however, radiologic or nephrosonographic studies are used to demonstrate papillary necrosis. Analgesic nephropathy occurs mostly in middle-aged women who have a history of personality disorders and chronic headache. Because many persons with the disease deny abuse of analgesics, testing the urine for metabolites of phenacetin and/or aspirin can be useful.

Symptoms of the disease occur rather late and include physical indications of premature aging, a brownish discoloration of the skin, inability to concentrate the urine, sterile leukocyturia, anemia and metabolic acidosis. Renal colic may be caused by the passage of papillary fragments. After discontinuation of analgesic usage, renal function may remain stable for many years or even improve.

Radiologic Features: Radiologic studies reveal bilateral papillary necrosis in different stages of development. Even though the pyelographic signs of total or partial papillary necrosis (namely, ring shadows, medullary cavities and calcifications) are well known, it should be pointed out that papillary necrosis in analgesic nephropathy may occur without sloughing, a process called in situ necrosis. In such cases, the radiologic diagnosis may be difficult or impossible.

Macroscopic Findings: In the early stages of the disease, both kidneys are of normal size. Their surfaces are smooth. Close inspection shows yellow-white streaks in the papillae, mainly at their tips. In advanced stages, the kidneys are shrunken and about equal in size. Their surfaces display sagittal bars of hypertrophic areas that correspond to the columns of Bertini; these bars alternate with retracted cortical areas that overlie the necrotic papillae. On cut surface, the most striking findings are alterations in the papillae. Almost all papillae in both kidneys show evidence of different stages of necrosis. The necrotic papillae have a dense consistency and a brownish discoloration. Entire papillae or parts of them may have become sequestered. The remaining medulla is concave with multiple clefts. The renal pelvis and calices are not affected.

Light Microscopic Findings: Papillary necrosis is the hallmark of analgesic nephropathy. There are three morphologic stages of papillary change:

Early changes are confined to the papillae and the inner medulla. They consist of marked thickening of the basement membranes of the loops of Henle and accompanying capillaries as well as changes in the matrix of the medulla. There is patchy necrosis of cells of the loops of Henle and of interstitial cells, but the collecting ducts that run through these areas remain unaffected.

In intermediate, or partial, papillary necrosis, the necrotic areas are confluent and unevenly distributed. They extend up to the corticomedullary junction. Collecting ducts also are involved. Few inflammatory cells are observed around the necrotic areas. At this stage, the first changes appear in the cortex; the changes consist of focal areas of atrophic tubules, with interstitial fibrosis overlying the necrotic papillae.

Advanced, or total, papillary necrosis involves the papillae as well as the medulla. The confluent necrosis displays a zone of demarcation at the corticomedullary junction, and remarkably few inflammatory cells are seen at the boundary between necrotic and viable tissue. The papillae may remain in situ, show incomplete detachment with cystic clefts at the demarcation zone or become sloughed off. The necrotic tissue often is calcified and may even be ossified.

In advanced papillary necrosis, there is an extending tubular atrophy in the cortex as well as diffuse interstitial fibrosis with few inflammatory cells, mainly lymphocytes and plasma cells. This so-called chronic interstitial nephritis develops after papillary necrosis and seems to be a consequence of it. The glomeruli are crowded because of tubular atrophy, but they remain unaffected for a long time. In later stages, periglomerular fibrosis and focal-segmental glomerulosclerosis and hyalinosis appear. Focal-segmental glomerulosclerosis is especially pronounced in cases with proteinuria and progressive renal failure.

Electron Microscopic Findings: Electron microscopy of early changes in the inner medullary zone shows a marked concentric lamellar thickening of the basement membranes of the loops of Henle and accompanying capillaries. Their lumina are narrowed, and the epithelial and endothelial cells display degenerative changes. The interstitial cells lose their processes, and autophagic vacuoles appear in their cytoplasm.

Immunofluorescence Microscopic Findings: No immunopathologic characteristics or mechanisms have been demonstrated in analgesic nephropathy by fluorescence microscopy.

Changes in Renal Pelvis and Ureter. Highly characteristic (or even pathognomonic) for analgesic nephropathy is a homogeneous thickening of the walls of the capillaries just beneath the transitional epithelium (urothelium) in the pelvic, ureteral and bladder mucosa. This "capillary sclerosis" is best seen in periodic acid-Schiff-stained sections. Electron microscopy demonstrates thickening of the basement membranes; the thickening is caused by numerous concentrically arranged lamellae and a variety of particulate and vesicular structures in between the lamellae.

Brownish discoloration of the mucosal membranes of the lower urinary tract is a frequent finding in analgesic nephropathy. It seems to be related to capillary sclerosis.

The association between analgesic abuse and transitional cell carcinoma of the pelvis and ureter has been well established.

Pathogenesis: Although the descriptive pathologic features of analgesic nephropathy are fairly well established, the pathogenesis remains a subject of controversy. It is not known whether the initiating event in the development of papillary necrosis is direct damage to tubular cells, interstitial cells and the matrix or whether vascular changes are the precipitating event. Available evidence indicates that one or more of the metabolites of mixed analgesic compounds may have direct toxic actions.

Lithium Nephropathy

Lithium is used in the management of manic-depressive psychosis and, occasionally, other psychiatric disorders. On rare occasions, it causes acute renal failure, but the pathogenesis of this effect is unknown. Chronic effects of lithium administration include polyuria, decreased ability to concentrate urine, nephrogenic diabetes insipidus, tubulo-interstitial nephritis and, in rare cases, renal failure. Tubulo-interstitial abnormalities include tubular dilatation, tubular atrophy, interstitial fibrosis around affected tubules and, in some instances, glomerular sclerosis. There have been reports of a specific tubular lesion, namely, epithelial cell enlargement and vacuolation of cytoplasm in the distal tubules and collecting ducts, as well as microcyst formation. Scanning electron microscopy reveals that the enlarged cells in the collecting ducts are mainly light cells; the dark cells are practically unaffected.

Chloroethyl-cyclohexyl Nitrosourea (CCNU) Nephropathy

Nitrosourea compounds, such as CCNU (chloroethyl-cyclohexyl nitrosourea) and methyl-CCNU are used in the management of neoplastic disorders. When given in large doses, they may lead to chronic tubulo-interstitial disease and renal failure, probably by causing tubular necrosis and atrophy.

Table II Drug-Induced Renal Injury with
Suggested Mechanisms

Acetaminophen	Tubulotoxic	Cyclosporin A	Tubulotoxic
Acetylsalicylic acid	Tubulotoxic	Diflunisal	Immunoallergic
Adriamycin	Tubulotoxic	Dimethylchlor-tetracycline	Tubulotoxic
Allopurinol*	Immunoallergic		
Aminoglycosides (Amikacin, capreomycin, gentamicin, kanamycin, neomycin, paromomycin, streptomycin, tobramycin, vancomycin, viomycin)	Tubulotoxic	Fenoprofen	Immunoallergic
		Furosemide	Immunoallergic
		Glafenine	Immunoallergic
		Indomethacin	Immunoallergic
		6-Mercaptopurine	Immunoallergic
		Mercurials	Tubulotoxic
		Methicillin	Immunoallergic
		Methotrexate	Tubulotoxic
		Methylphenidate	Tubulotoxic
		Minocycline	Immunoallergic
		Nafcillin	Immunoallergic
Amphotericin B	Tubulotoxic	Naproxen	Immunoallergic
Ampicillin	Immunoallergic	Oxacillin	Immunoallergic
Azathioprine	Immunoallergic	para-Aminosalicylic acid	Immunoallergic
Bacitracin	Tubulotoxic		
Bismuth	Tubulotoxic	Penicillin G	Immunoallergic
Boric acid	Tubulotoxic	Phenazone	Immunoallergic
Busulfan	Tubulotoxic	Phenindione	Immunoallergic
Calcium versinate	Tubulotoxic	Phenobarbital	Immunoallergic
Carbenicillin	Immunoallergic	Phenylbutazone	Tubulotoxic, immunoallergic
Carbimazole	Tubulotoxic		
Cephaloridine	Tobulotoxic, immunoallergic	Phenytoin	
		Polymyxin B	Tubulotoxic, immunoallergic
Cephalothin	Tubulotoxic, immunoallergic		
		Rifampicin	Immunoallergic
Cephalexin	Immunoallergic	Sulfonamides	Tubulotoxic, immunoallergic
cis-Platinum	Tubulotoxic		
Clofibrate	Immunoallergic	Thiazides	Immunoallergic
Chloramphenicol	Immunoallergic	Tolmetin	Immunoallergic
Colistin	Tubulotoxic	? Uroradiographic contrast media	Tubulotoxic
Co-trimoxazole	Immunoallergic		

*Underlined drugs frequently induce acute tubulo-interstitial nephritis.

Drug-Induced Tubulo-interstitial Nephritis
Acute Tubulotoxic Injury

Fig. 5-1 Acetaminophen. Fatty degeneration of tubules in a child after administration of high doses of the drug. (osmium fixation, hematoxylin and eosin, ×430)

Fig. 5-2 Methylphenidate. Acute renal failure after administration of the drug. Tubular necrosis and interstitial inflammation are present. (hematoxylin and eosin, ×270)

Fig. 5-3 Busulfan. Tubular cells showing large hyperchromatic nuclei. No serious functional disturbances were observed. (hematoxylin and eosin, ×430)

Drug-Induced Hypersensitivity Tubulo-interstitial Nephritis

Fig. 5-4 Methicillin. Diffuse interstitial inflammation. (hematoxylin and eosin, ×110)

Fig. 5-5 Allopurinol. Interstitial inflammation with focal tubular destruction. (hematoxylin and eosin, ×160)

Fig. 5-6 Iodine. Severe tubulo-interstitial inflammation with tubulorrhexis after administration of iodochlorhydroxyquin. (hematoxylin and eosin, ×270)

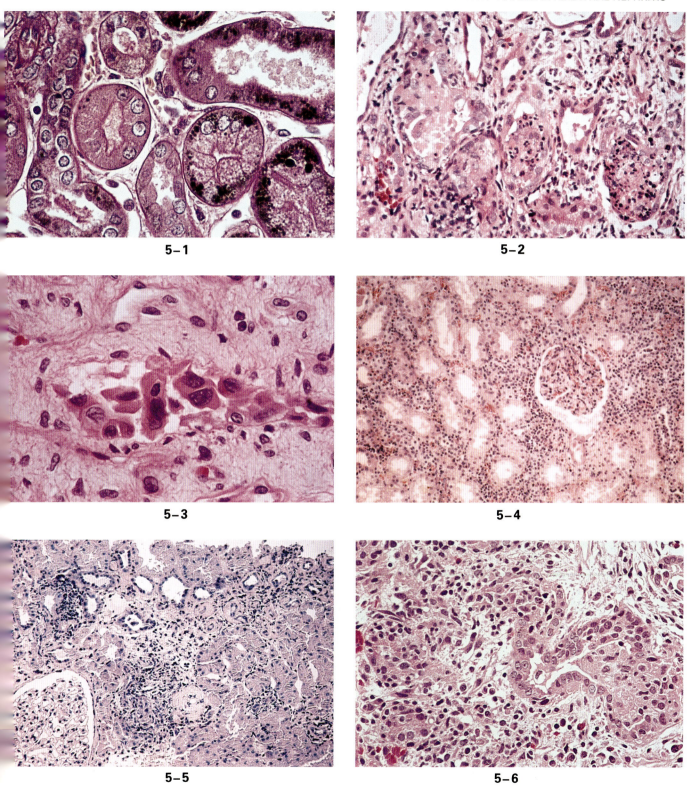

5-1

5-2

5-3

5-4

5-5

5-6

Drug-Induced Hypersensitivity Tubulo-interstitial Nephritis

Fig. 5-7   Erythromycin. Granulomatous interstitial inflammation with giant cells and many eosinophils. (hematoxylin and eosin, ×220)

Fig. 5-8   Erthyromycin. Peritubular deposits of complement (C3) in the same case as in Figure 5-7. (fluorescence microscopy, ×270)

Fig. 5-9   Erthyromycin. Cervical lymph node showing sarcoid-like granulomatous reaction. Same case as in Figure 5-8. Patient had no evidence of sarcoidosis. Lymphadenopathy resolved concurrently with disappearance of renal symptoms. (hematoxylin and eosin, ×270)

Analgesic Nephropathy

Fig. 5-10   Analgesic nephropathy, early stage. "In situ" papillary necrosis in a case of long-standing phenacetin abuse.

Fig. 5-11   Histologic section showing ischemic necrosis of medulla and preservation of cortex. There is practically no inflammatory reaction. (hematoxylin and eosin, ×10)

Fig. 5-12   Necrosis of epithelium of loops of Henle. Collecting ducts and blood vessels are preserved. (hematoxylin and eosin, ×270)

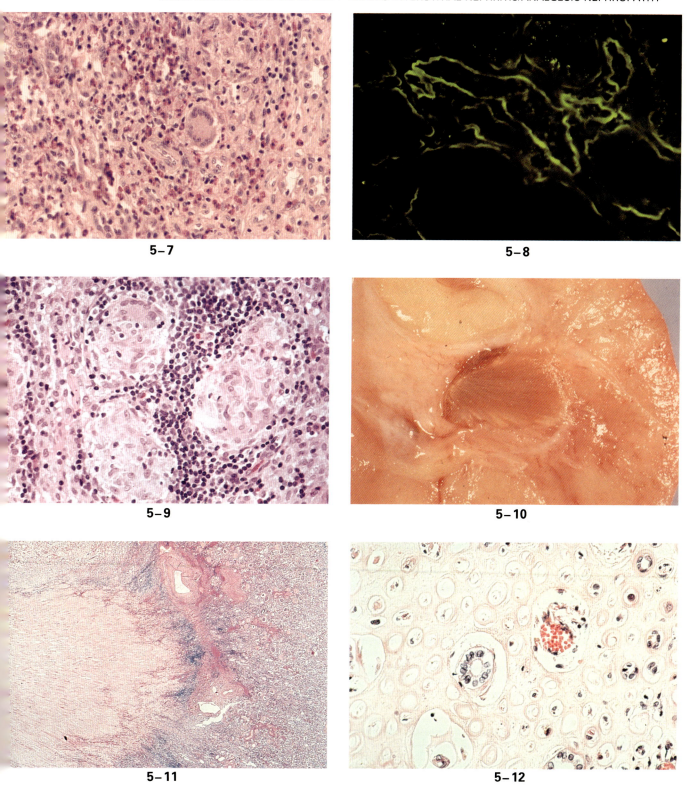

5–7

5–8

5–9

5–10

5–11

5–12

Analgesic Nephropathy

Fig. 5-13 Analgesic nephropathy. Marked thickening of basement membranes of loops of Henle. (periodic acid-Schiff/alcian blue, ×270)

Fig. 5-14 Analgesic nephropathy, late stage. Papillary necrosis with dark brown coloration and segmentation of papillae.

Fig. 5-15 Analgesic nephropathy, late stage. Papillary necrosis with beginning of sloughing. (hematoxylin and eosin, ×10)

Fig. 5-16 Analgesic nephropathy, late stage. Atrophic kidney showing necrosis, sclerosis and brown discoloration of papillae and of pelvic and ureteral mucosa.

Fig. 5-17 Analgesic nephropathy. Dilatation of the calix, loss of papillae, necrosis of inner medulla and scarring of overlying cortex. (hematoxylin and eosin, ×3)

Fig. 5-18 Small blood vessels in pelvic submucosa showing marked capillary sclerosis ("microangiopathy"). (periodic acid-Schiff, ×430)

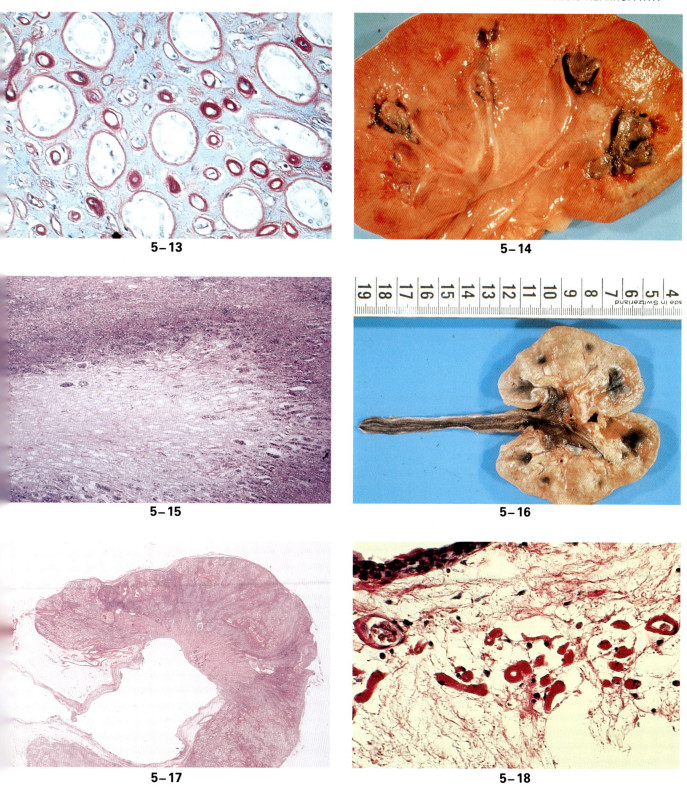

5–13

5–14

5–15

5–16

5–17

5–18

Analgesic Nephropathy

Fig. 5-19 Schematic presentation of radiologic appearance of analgesic nephropathy.

Fig. 5-20 Analgesic nephropathy. Focal segmental glomerulosclerosis in a patient with severe proteinuria. (periodic acid-Schiff, ×270)

Fig. 5-21 Analgesic nephropathy. Papillary transitional cell carcinoma of pelvis.

Chronic Lithium Nephropathy

Fig. 5-22 Lithium nephropathy. Numerous small cysts in cortex.

Fig. 5-23 Lithium nephropathy. Tubular atrophy and interstitial fibrosis with areas of tubular dilatation. (hematoxylin and eosin, ×110)

Fig. 5-24 Localized areas of tubular fibrosis. Sclerotic glomerulus is seen in left lower corner. (picro-Sirius, ×45)

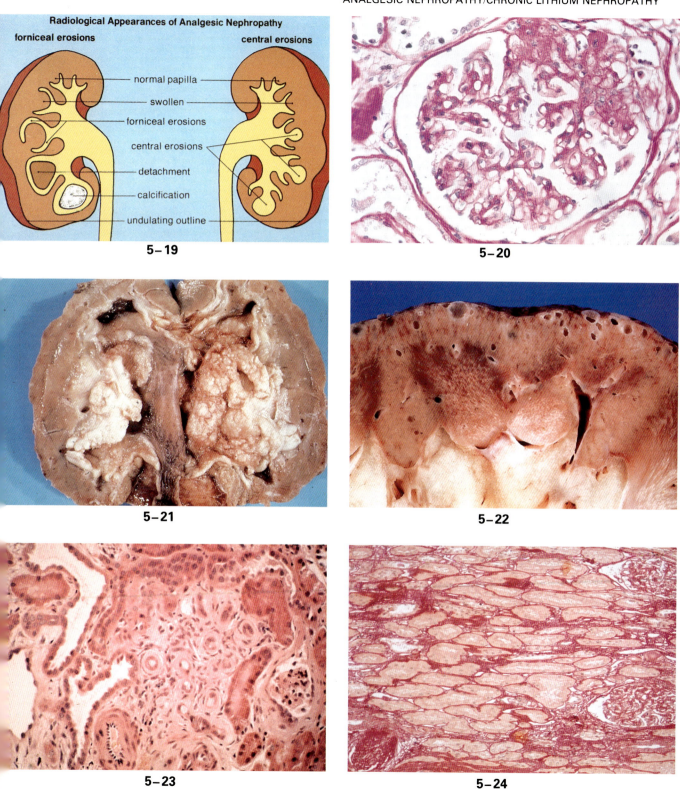

Radiological Appearances of Analgesic Nephropathy

forniceal erosions

central erosions

- normal papilla
- swollen
- forniceal erosions
- central erosions
- detachment
- calcification
- undulating outline

5–19

5–20

5–21

5–22

5–23

5–24

Drug-Induced Tubulotoxic Injury

Fig. 5-25 Tubulotoxic damage after administration of methylphenidate. Cell in center shows marked pyknosis of mitochondria and condensation of cytoplasm. (electron micrograph, ×4200)

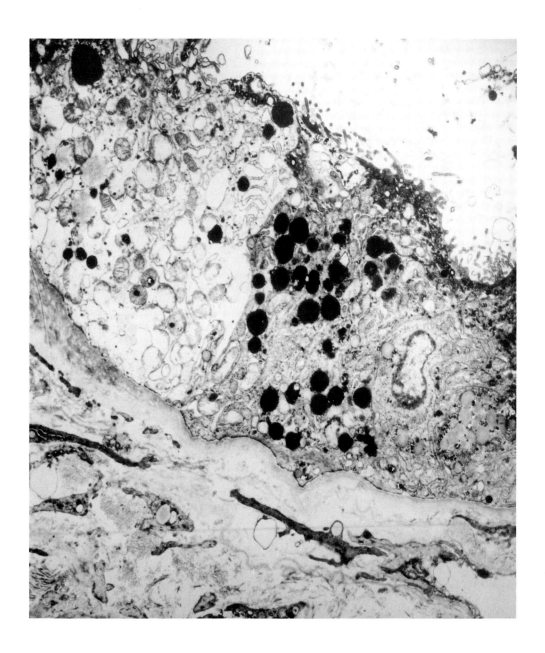

Drug-Induced Tubulotoxic Injruy

Fig. 5-26 Gentamicin toxicity. Tubular cell containing myelin-like bodies in lyso-somes. (electron micrograph, ×7500)

Fig. 5-27 Gentamicin toxicity. High magnification showing fine structure of mye-lin-like bodies. (electron micrograph, ×20,000)

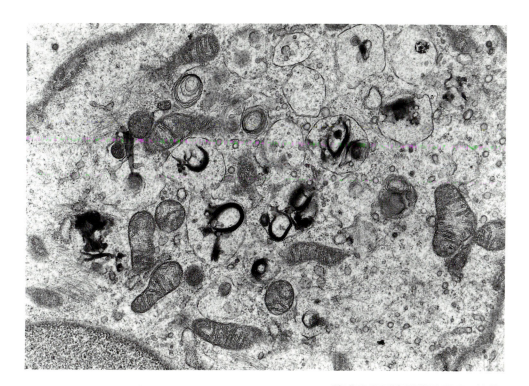

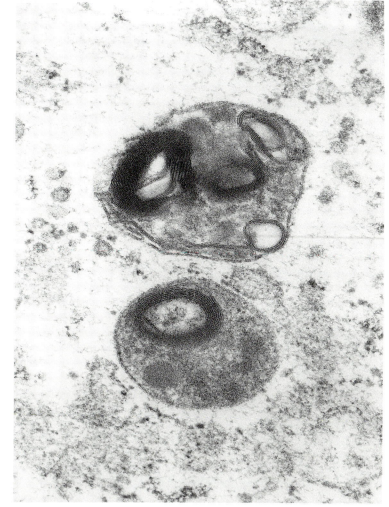

Analgesic Nephropathy

Fig. 5-28 Analgesic nephropathy with papillary necrosis. Retrograde pyelogram showing various changes: "Lobster claw" deformity, large papillary cavity with extension between pyramid and column of Bertin (thick arrow); small, rounded papillary cavity connecting with calix in upper middle pole (thin arrow); and pointed, narrow papilla, probably "necrosis in situ" in lowermost calix (arrowhead).

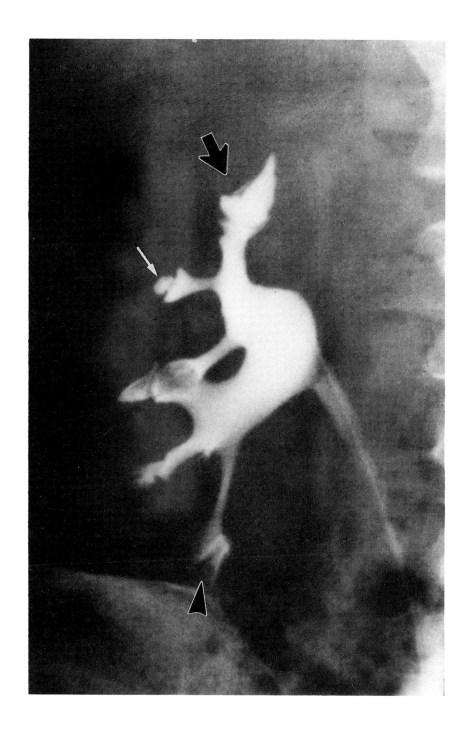

Analgesic Nephropathy/Chronic Lithium Nephropathy

Fig. 5-29 Analgesic nephropathy. Capillary in ureter showing marked thickening of wall by multiple layers of basement membrane. (electron micrograph, ×3800)

Fig. 5-30 Cortical collecting duct from lithium-treated rat. Bulging light cells form hobnail-like projections into lumen. (scanning electron micrograph ×1000)

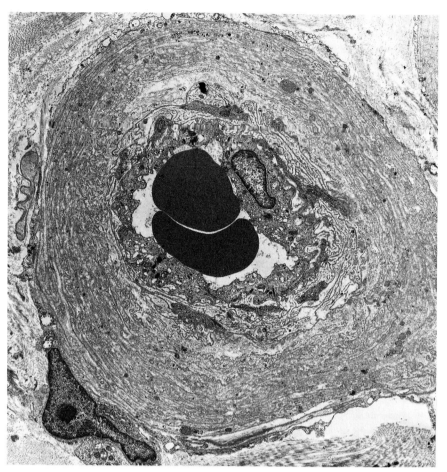

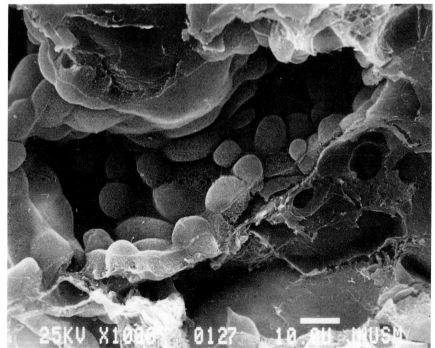

Tubulo-interstitial Nephritis Associated with Immune Disorders

Tubulo-interstitial Nephritis Associated with Immune Disorders

This group of renal diseases is characterized by morphologic or functional changes, or both, involving the tubules (usually the proximal convoluted) and interstitium. For each disease in this group, the pathogenesis has been convincingly or tentatively ascribed to a hypersensitivity reaction. Some tubulo-interstitial nephritides are associated with immunologically mediated primary glomerular diseases, whereas others are restricted to the tubulo-interstitium.

Because various immunologic mechanisms utilize similar mediators to produce tissue damage, it is not surprising that use of histologic findings alone to differentiate the various immunologically mediated tubulo-interstitial nephritides is of scarce help in their classification. Studies performed in laboratory animals have shown that various types of tubulo-interstitial nephritis may be experimentally induced by one or more mechanisms of hypersensitivity. Identification of pertinent etiologic factors would be the most sound basis for the classification of these diseases in human beings. The etiologic basis, however, is frequently unknown. Therefore, at present, the best classification may be one that takes into account basic immunopathogenetic mechanisms as well as etiologic factors. Table I (see p. 2) represents an attempt to classify immunologically mediated tubulo-interstitial nephritides in human beings in a schematic manner. It should be kept in mind, however, that during the course of such diseases, more than one pathogenetic mechanism can operate concomitantly or at sequential intervals.

Tubulo-interstitial Nephritis Induced by Antibodies Reacting with Tubular Antigens (antitubular basement membrane disease)

There is conclusive evidence that antitubular basement membrane antibody-mediated disease occurs in human beings, but it is a rare entity. Antibody to tubular basement membranes is evidenced by linear deposits of IgG and C3 along the membranes. Moreover, eluates of renal tissues contain antibodies that react with glomerular basement membranes, tubular basement membranes and, sometimes, pulmonary basement membranes. These findings indicate that autoantibodies are directed against shared antigenic determinants within these basement membranes. In renal allografts, the tubular basement membrane antibodies may be alloantibodies. In this setting, they react only with the graft and not with the kidney of the recipient.

Anti-TBM nephritis can occur in the following conditions:

Antiglomerular Basement Membrane Glomerulonephritis (Goodpasture's syndrome)

In about one-half of patients with antiglomerular basement membrane glomerulonephritis, or Goodpasture's syndrome, antibodies react with the basement membranes of the proximal convoluted tubules. Comparative studies performed in patients with this form of glomerulonephritis, associated or not associated with tubular basement membrane antibodies, suggest that such antibodies contribute to the genesis of tubulo-interstitial lesions.

Immune Complex Glomerulonephritis

Linear staining for IgG along basement membranes of the proximal convoluted tubules may be found in a few patients with membranous glomerulonephritis or poststreptococcal glomerulonephritis. Occasionally, antitubular basement membrane antibody may be found in the serum. In addition to nephrotic syndrome, some such patients have glycosuria, aminoaciduria and moderate to severe interstitial and tubular lesions.

Drug Induced

Tubulo-interstitial nephritis associated with linear deposits of IgG along tubular basement membranes develops in a small percentage of patients who receive methicillin, cloxacillin or phenytoin.

Idiopathic

There has been one report of a patient with severe tubulo-interstitial nephritis, linear deposits of IgG along the tubular basement membranes, circulating antibodies to the tubular basement membranes and renal tubular acidosis.

Renal Allografts

The tubular basement membranes of the proximal convoluted tubules contain alloantigens. When a tubular basement membrane alloantigen-positive kidney is transplanted into an alloantigen-negative recipient, formation of antitubular basement membrane alloantibodies can occur. The alloantibodies react only with tubular basement membranes of the graft. There is no firm evidence that the alloantibodies can induce tubulo-interstitial lesions. Occasionally, renal allografts may elicit the formation of tubular basement membrane autoantibodies that react with the tubular basement membranes of the graft as well as with those of the recipient's kidneys, if the native kidneys are still in situ.

Microscopic Findings In Antitubular Basement Membrane Disease: Interstitial infiltration with polymorphonuclear leukocytes, especially along tubular basement membranes, and edema are seen in the initial stage, which is encountered rarely because renal biopsies usually are not available. While the disease progresses, severe infiltration with lymphocytes, monocytes, macrophages and plasma cells becomes evident. In rare cases, large numbers of epithelioid and giant cells are seen in the interstitium. The giant cells do not appear to be in contact with tubular basement membranes, and phagocytosis of membrane fragments is not observed. Other characteristics of antitubular basement membrane nephritis are exudative and proliferative changes of the tubules. Polymorphonuclear leukocytes, lymphocytes and monocytes penetrate between epithelial cells, and focal destruction of tubular basement membranes is frequently observed. In proximal and distal convoluted tubules, proliferating epithelial cells partially or completely obliterate the tubular lumina. Some lumina contain "casts" formed by necrotic epithelial nuclei. In later stages, there is widespread thickening and "splitting" of tubular basement membranes, tubular atrophy and interstitial fibrosis.

Immunofluorescence Microscopic Findings: The most distinctive immunocytochemical feature in all the above forms of tubulo-interstitial nephritis is linear deposition of IgG along basement membranes of the proximal convoluted tubules. Similar deposits of C3 are found in about 50% of patients with antiglomerular/antitubular basement membrane nephritis.

IgG eluted from nephritic kidneys reacts with tubular basement membranes of normal human kidney in vitro. Occasionally, antitubular basement membrane antibodies, with similar reactivity, are detectable in the sera of such patients.

Functional abnormalities are not well known because the disease is rare in its pure form. When associated with antiglomerular basement membrane glomerulonephritis, the role of tubular basement membrane antibody is difficult to assess. In some patients, however, abnormalities that are characteristic of proximal tubular acidosis, with or without Fanconi's syndrome, are observed.

Tubulo-interstitial Nephritis Induced by Autologous or Exogenous Antigen-Antibody (immune) Complexes

Immune complex tubulo-interstitial nephritis is observed in a number of clinical settings. It is evidenced by granular fluorescence along tubular basement membranes and in the interstitium. The clinical settings in which this disease has been observed most frequently are described below.

Systemic Lupus Erythematosus

Tubulo-interstitial nephritis associated with local deposits of immunoglobulin and complement is found in about 30% to 60% of patients with severe, diffuse, proliferative and exudative lupus glomerulonephritis. Granular deposits of immunoglobulins and C3 are seen along peritubular capillaries, basement membranes of proximal convoluted tubules and in the interstitium. Infiltrates of inflammatory cells, fibrosis and tubular cell damage also are present, suggesting that the immune deposits may have pathogenetic implications. In a few patients, DNA products have been demonstrated in immune deposits. This finding is consistent with the interpretation that immune deposits contain immune complexes. Some patients with tubulo-interstitial lesions have glycosuria with a normal blood glucose level. Other patients with normal glomerular function have alterations of renal acidification, concentrating ability and secretion of potassium. These tubular abnormalities could be related to tubulo-interstitial lesions. Three patients with lupus associated acute or chronic tubulo-interstitial nephritis but without or with mild glomerulonephritis have been described.

Mixed Cryoglobulinemia

Patients with mixed cryoglobulinemia and glomerulonephritis may have mild or severe tubulo-interstitial nephritis associated with granular immune deposits in the interstitium or along basement membranes of the proximal convoluted tubules. The pathogenetic role of the immune deposits, which presumably contain immune complexes, is not known. It should be stressed that patients with mixed cryoglobulinemia may have severe tubulo-interstitial nephritis without local immune deposits. Thus, it is conceivable that in conditions characterized by cryoglobulinemia, tubulo-interstitial lesions may be induced by a variety of pathogenetic mechanisms.

Bacterial Immune Complex Glomerulonephritis

Tubulo-interstitial nephritis can occur in patients with severe, acute forms of bacterial glomerulonephritis seemingly due to immune complex mechanisms. In this category may fall a few patients with acute bacterial endocarditis in whom large amounts of immune deposits are found in the interstitium, peritubular capillaries and tubular basement membranes. The interstitium contains infiltrates of mononuclear cells, polymorphonuclear leukocytes and plasma cells. These tubulo-interstitial lesions usually are reversible if the etiologic agent can be eradicated by antibiotic treatment.

Sjögren's Syndrome

Some patients with Sjögren's syndrome have glomerulonephritis with granular immune deposits, tubulo-interstitial nephritis or both. Such patients have distinctive abnormalities of tubular function. Despite the high frequency of these changes, progressive renal failure and uremia are seldom the cause of death. The most characteristic renal lesion is a chronic tubulo-interstitial nephritis with interstitial infiltrates of lymphocytes and plasma cells, severe peritubular fibrosis and tubular atrophy. The cortex and the medulla can be affected. Ribbon-like or coarse granular deposits of IgG and C3, which correspond to the dense deposits seen on electron microscopy, can be found in the tubular basement membranes. Deposits of IgG may be present in the cytoplasm of the plasma cells. These immunopathologic findings are by no means constant, and several patients with Sjögren's syndrome have had tubulo-interstitial nephritis without renal immune deposits.

The most frequent functional abnormality is impairment of the ability to concentrate and to acidify the urine. The defect of urinary concentration may be so marked as to produce a picture of nephrogenic diabetes insipidus. Other abnormalities of tubular function include partial or complete tubular acidosis, aminoaciduria and impairment of the ability to absorb phosphorus and uric acid.

The etiologic basis and the pathogenesis of Sjögren's syndrome are unknown.

Hypocomplementemic Glomerulonephritis

This disease is characterized by recurrent urticaria, cutaneous vasculitis, hypocomplementemia and glomerulonephritis. On occasion, immune complex deposits are found along tubular basement membranes.

Renal Allografts

The most frequent form of tubulo-interstitial nephritis seen in renal allografts is that associated with cell-mediated rejection. However, in about 5% of patients with long-standing renal allografts, coarse granular deposits of IgG, IgM and/or C3 are found along basement membranes of the proximal convoluted tubules. Mild infiltrates of mononuclear cells and areas of fibrosis can be observed in the interstitium; tubular atrophy also is seen. A pathogenetic relationship between tubular immune deposits and tubulo-interstitial lesions has not been established. In rabbits with renal allografts, similar lesions may occur as a consequence of in situ formation of immune complexes. Such complexes contain antigens released from the cytoplasm of tubular cells. The composition of the granular immune deposits found in tubular basement membranes of human renal allografts is not known.

Tubulo-interstitial Changes in Renal Allografts

A variety of changes may be seen in transplanted kidneys, involving any or all of its structural components. Glomerular alterations are described in the volume on glomerular diseases; vascular alterations are presented in the volume on vascular diseases.

Tubular and interstitial injury can be generally ascribed to four pathogenetic mechanisms: pretransplant ischemia; direct damage induced by the immune response of the host, mainly the cellular type of rejection; ischemia due to vascular injury, most often vascular rejection but, on occasion, a technical failure of anastomosis; and infection, either acquired shortly after operation, especially if there is partial obstruction of the site of ureteral anastomosis, or rejection injury of the ureter (ascending infection) or as part of disseminated infection promoted by immunosuppression. All these changes may coexist or occur sequentially, and they are not always easy to distinguish from each other, particularly when only a small biopsy specimen is available for examination.

Pretransplant ischemic changes may be manifest by vacuolation and granulation of tubular cells or, with prolonged ischemia, as fairly diffuse, rather bland necrosis, accompanied on occasion by sparse infiltration by small lymphocytes and polymorphonuclear leukocytes. At a later stage, cellular regeneration may be noted, indicating the likelihood of functional recovery.

Cellular rejection first appears shortly after transplantation (two to 10 days) but may occur at any time during the life of the transplant. Patchy, mainly perivascular but occasionally diffuse, infiltrates consist of lymphocytes, plasma cells, large mononuclear cells (immunoblasts) and, sometimes, a small number of polymorphonuclear leukocytes. The interstitial tissue is characteristically edematous, leading to separation of the tubules. Edema often persists even after the inflammatory exudate is reduced or eliminated by immunosuppressive therapy. More severe tubular damage may occur, with necrosis of cells and disruption of basement membranes, but when inflammation is reduced, the tubules usually regenerate.

Tubulo-interstitial changes that accompany acute vascular rejection vary from large infarcts to small patches of necrosis. Even without obvious necrosis, there often are more or less extensive hemorrhages into interstitial tissue. Focal infiltrates of inflammatory cells also may be found; the infiltrates contain lymphocytes, plasma cells and polymorphonuclear leukocytes, the latter being most noticeable along the edges of necrosis. In chronic vascular rejection, there is progressive contraction of the renal parenchyma, tubular atrophy and destruction, large amounts of loose fibrous tissue and scattering of chronic inflammatory cells.

Unless the causative organism is demonstrated in sections or by culture, infection of the renal graft may be particularly difficult to recognize. Polymorphonuclear leukocytes in the tubular lumina, pus casts and a large number of polymorphonuclear leukocytes in the peritubular connective tissue are suggestive but not necessarily diagnostic. It sometimes is necessary to treat a patient on the basis of clinical suspicion.

Tubulo-interstitial Nephritis Induced by, or Associated with, Cell-Mediated Hypersensitivity

Several observations indicate that cell-mediated hypersensitivity may have an important role in the pathogenesis of some forms of tubulo-interstitial nephritis. 1) The disease can occur during the course of other diseases (tuberculosis, leprosy, measles and other bacterial, viral and parasitic infections) that are characterized by cell-mediated hypersensitivity. 2) There is a pronounced mononuclear cell infiltrate in the renal interstitium and an absence of circulating antibodies that react with renal antigens or of immune deposits in tubulo-interstitial structures. 3) Lymphocyte hypersensitivity has been demonstrated to certain antigens (usually drugs) that have been implicated in the development of the disease. 4) Immunofluorescence studies have shown that most cells that have infiltrated the interstitium are stimulated T lymphocytes. 5) Tubulo-interstitial nephritis in human beings is similar to certain experimentally induced forms of the disease, in the sense that they are characterized by lymphocyte hypersensitivity to the eliciting antigen; also, in these forms, it is possible to transfer the lesion from a nephritic to a healthy animal by use of cells but not serum.

It must be emphasized that although the histologic appearance of mononuclear cell infiltration is frequently consistent with a cell-mediated reaction, this observation can hardly be considered a proof, especially since it appears that antibodies or immune complexes may induce, at some stages, a predominantly mononuclear cell infiltrate. Therefore, a demonstration that some forms of tubulo-interstitial nephritis are mediated by cellular hypersensitivity is, most frequently, lacking. To confirm this hypothesis, we must first learn to document clearly cell-mediated immunity in human tubulo-interstitial diseases. Then, the latter mechanism may prove to be more important than either immune complex or antitulular basement antibodies. Furthermore, it may be that cell-mediated hypersensitivity is elicited by antigens that are released from renal tissues damaged by antibodies or immune complexes. According to this interpretation, cellular mechanisms could cooperate with antibodies or immune complexes in the development and, especially, in the progression of tubulo-interstitial injury.

Tubulo-interstitial Nephritis Induced by Immediate (IgE Type) Hypersensitivity

Drug-induced acute tubulo-interstitial nephritis appears to be due to a hypersensitivity reaction. Patients who are known to have hypersensitivity to a certain drug, on exposure to the drug, may suffer from acute tubulo-interstitial nephritis. Methicillin, rifampicin and phenindione have been implicated most frequently (Table III). Other offending drugs include sulfonamides, various types of penicillin, thiazides, furosemide, allopurinol and fenoprofen. Some reports have mentioned combinations of drugs.

The most accurate clinical information concerns hypersensitivity to methicillin. The disease, which may occur at any age, develops about 10 to 15 days after the beginning of drug administration and is characterized by fever, hematuria and mild proteinuria, which occurs in 70% of patients.. There is no correlation between dosage and the occurrence of tubulo-interstitial nephritis. Transient eosinophilia is found in 80% and skin rash in about 25% of patients. Eosinophils can be detected in urinary sediments. From 20% to 50% of patients have oliguria or anuria in combination with azotemia, which is most severe in older patients. Other abnormalities of renal function include distal renal tubular acidosis, sodium-losing nephropathy and potassium retention. Signs of renal failure usually are transient, and urinary abnormalities disappear a few days after discontinuation of methicillin administration. However, in older patients, elevations of the creatinine level and urea nitrogen may persist for long periods. The effectiveness of corticosteroid treatment is a subject of debate. Likewise, there is no firm evidence that reexposure of allergic patients to methicillin or cross-reacting drugs involves a greater risk for the development of tubulo-interstitial nephritis. A few reports have noted the simultaneous occurrence of tubulo-interstitial nephritis and the foot-process type of minimal glomerular disease with nephrotic syndrome in patients receiving nonsteroidal antiinflammatory agents, such as fenoprofen.

The study of renal tissue obtained by biopsy during the early stages of disease reveals focal interstitial infiltration by mononuclear cells, mainly lymphocytes and monocytes. Basophils and eosinophils often are present, sometimes in high numbers and with aspects of degranulation. By means of electron microscopy, granules released from such cells can be observed in the interstitium. Infiltrates are most evident in the cortex. Diffuse interstitial edema and a variable degree of tubular cell degeneration and regeneration also are seen. In a few patients, epithelioid and giant cells, forming interstitial granulomas, have been described. In most reports concerned with acute tubulo-interstitial nephritis associated with penicillin G treatment, such lesions were associated with glomerular and vascular changes.

To prove that tubulo-interstitial nephritis is due to an immediate hypersensitivity reaction, the demonstration of the antigen and of IgE immunoglobulins in renal tissue is required. It is difficult, however, to fulfill these criteria because renal biopsies seldom are performed in the early stage of disease. There often is the possibility that fluorescein-conjugated antisera may bind nonspecifically to the surfaces of basophils or eosinophils. Furthermore, the antigen may be present in amounts undetectable by immunofluorescence, or it may no longer be present in interstitial tissue at the time of renal biopsy. Despite these limitations, the occurrence of a latent period, the lack of correlation with the drug dosage, the eosinophilia, the skin rash, the occasional history of drug hypersensitivity and of positive skin test reactions as well as the demonstration of degranulated basophils and eosinophils in renal tissue are strongly indicative of a hypersensitivity reaction mediated by reaginic antibodies. The IgE level may be increased and, in a few instances, IgE has been shown to display reactivity for methicillin. In several patients, linear deposits of IgG and C3 were observed along tubular basement membranes. In one patient treated with methicillin, linear deposits of IgG and C3 were found along tubular basement membranes, and antibody with reactivity for these membranes was found in the circulation. Furthermore, dimethoxyphenylpenicilloyl, the haptenic group of methicillin, was demonstrated by immunofluorescence along tubular basement membranes. These findings were interpreted as indicating that the drug hapten, which is secreted by proximal convoluted tubules, was bound to tubular basement membranes, thus stimulating production of antibodies to tubular basement membranes. In many other patients, however, linear deposition of IgG along tubular basement membranes was not observed.

In conclusion, the hypothesis that drug-induced acute tubulo-interstitial nephritis is due to immediate (IgE type) hypersensitivity or to antibodies to tubular basement membranes is attractive but remains to be proven. Penicillin components are found in renal interstitium and in tubular basement membranes of normal kidneys from patients treated with large doses of penicillin shortly before death. Therefore, it is conceivable that other mechanisms, such as cell-mediated hypersensitivity, might also have a role in the pathogenesis of drug-induced tubulo-interstitial nephritis.

In patients with acute tubulo-interstitial nephritis, foot process-type minimal glomerular disease and nephrotic syndrome due to administration of nonsteroidal antiinflammatory agents, such as fenoprofen, a T-cell hyperreactivity has been described. It is proposed that sensitized T cells, reacting with the antigen at the level of tubular, interstitial and glomerular structures, may release lymphokines and recruit the inflammatory cells that are responsible for the inflammatory reaction.

Table III Drugs Associated with the Development of Acute Hypersensitivity Reactions in the Kidneys*

Drugs most frequently associated with acute tubulo-interstitial nephritis
  Methicillin
  Rifampicin
  Phenindione
  Sulfonamides

Drugs less frequently associated with acute tubulo-interstitial nephritis
  Oxacillin
  Nafcillin
  Carbenicillin
  Cephalothin
  Cephalexin
  Glafenine
  Allopurinol
  Thiazides
  Furosemide
  Co-trimoxazole
  Phenylbutazone
  Phenazone
  Phenytoin
  Azathioprine
  Phenobarbital

Drugs occasionally associated with acute tubulo-interstitial nephritis and minimal glomerular disease
  Fenoprofen
  Naproxen
  Ampicillin

Drugs occasionally associated with acute tubulo-interstitial nephritis, vasculitis and glomerulonephritis
  Penicillin G

*See also Table II, p. 59.

Tubulo-interstitial Nephritis Induced by Antibody Reacting with Tubular Antigens

Fig. 6-1   Antibasement membrane-mediated nephritis. Severe interstitial inflammation with focal destruction of tubular basement membranes. (periodic acid-Schiff, ×220)

Fig. 6-2   Antibasement membrane-mediated nephritis. Linear deposits of human IgG in glomerular basement membranes and in basement membranes of proximal convoluted tubules. (fluorescence microscopy, ×430)

Renal Allograft

Fig. 6-3   Renal allograft. Acute transplant rejection showing interstitial infiltration by lymphocytes, immunoblasts and plasma cells. (hematoxylin and eosin, ×430)

Fig. 6-4   Cellular transplant rejection. Ribbon-like deposits of human IgG in tubular basement membranes. (fluorescence microscopy, ×430)

Tubulo-interstitial Nephritis Induced by Immune Complexes
Systemic Lupus Erythematosus

Fig. 6-5   Systemic lupus erythematosus. Patchy loss of tubules with interstitial fibrosis and inflammation. (periodic acid-Schiff/silver methenamine, ×270)

Fig. 6-6   Periodic acid-Schiff-positive peritubular and globular interstitial deposits. (periodic acid-Schiff, ×1100)

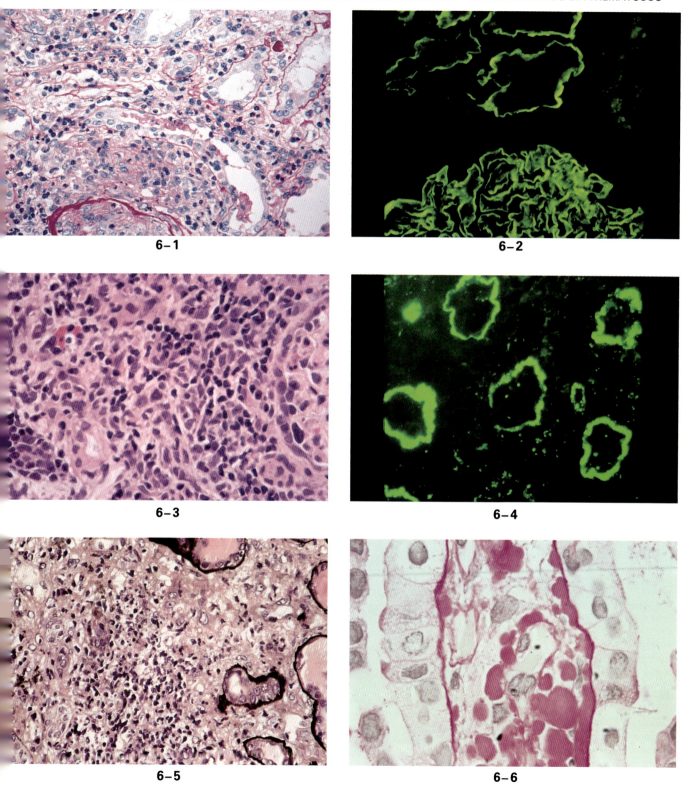

6–1

6–2

6–3

6–4

6–5

6–6

Tubulo-interstitial Nephritis Induced by Immune Complexes
Systemic Lupus Erythematosus

Fig. 6-7 Granular deposits of IgG along glomerular and tubular basement membranes. (fluorescence microscopy, ×430)

Hypocomplementemic Glomerulonephritis with Urticaria and Vasculitis

Fig. 6-8 Hypocomplementemic glomerulonephritis. Thickening of tubular basement membranes, interstitial edema and fibrosis. (periodic acid-Schiff, ×325)

Fig. 6-9 Same case as in Figure 6-8. Extensive deposits of IgG along tubular basement membranes. (fluorescence microscopy, ×325)

Sjögren's Syndrome

Fig. 6-10 Sjögren's syndrome. Extensive destruction of tubules with interstitial fibrosis and chronic inflammation. (periodic acid-Schiff, ×110)

Fig. 6-11 Granular and short linear deposits of IgG along tubular basement membranes. (fluorescence microscopy, ×430)

Tubulo-interstitial Nephritis Induced by Immediate (IgE Type) Hypersensitivity

Fig. 6-12 IgE-mediated tubulo-interstitial nephritis secondary to methicillin hypersensitivity. Interstitial infiltration by eosinophils with cellular degranulation and focal tubulorrhexis. (hematoxylin and eosin, ×400)

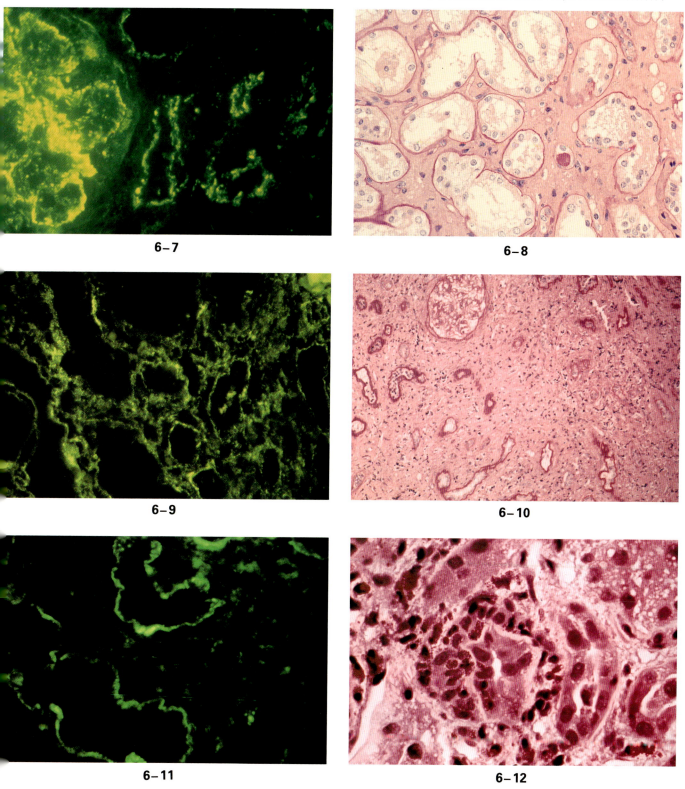

6–7

6–8

6–9

6–10

6–11

6–12

Systemic Lupus Erythematosus

Fig. 6-13 Systemic lupus erythematosus. Granular, electron-dense deposits within tubular basement membranes. (electron micrograph, ×10,000)

Fig. 6-14 Systemic lupus erythematosus. Globular, electron-dense deposits in renal interstitium. Compare with Figure 6-6. (electron micrograph, ×5000)

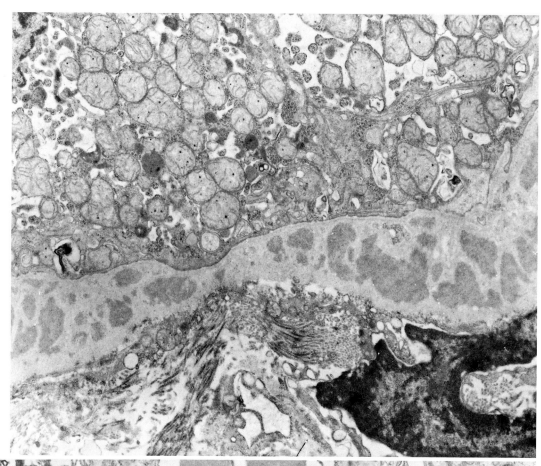
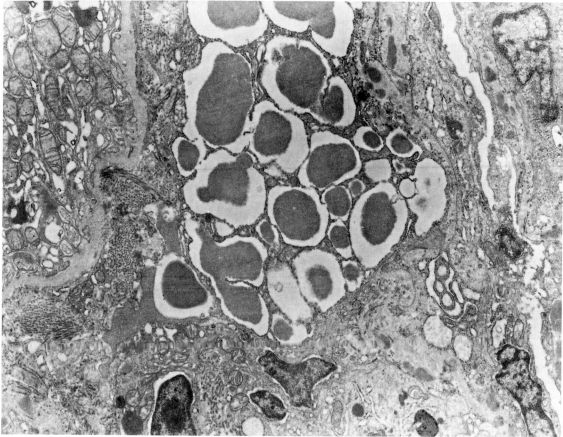

Systemic Lupus Erythematosus

Fig. 6-15 Systemic lupus erythematosus. Electron-dense deposits along wall of intertubular capillary. (electron micrograph, ×10,000)

Fig. 6-16 Hypocomplementemic glomerulonephritis and vasculitis. Small electron-dense deposits in tubular basement membranes. Same case as in Figure 6-8. (electron micrograph, ×10,000)

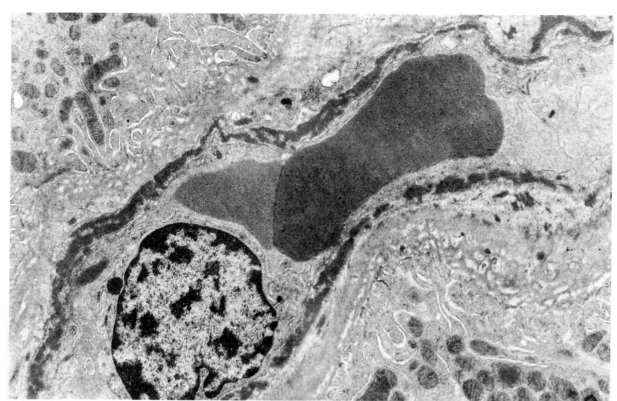

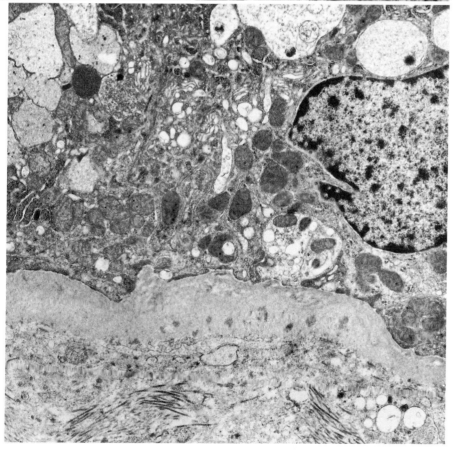

Sjögren's Syndrome

Fig. 6-17 Sjögren's syndrome. Granular, electron-dense deposits in tubular basement membranes. Same case as in Figure 6-10. (electron micrograph, ×8000)

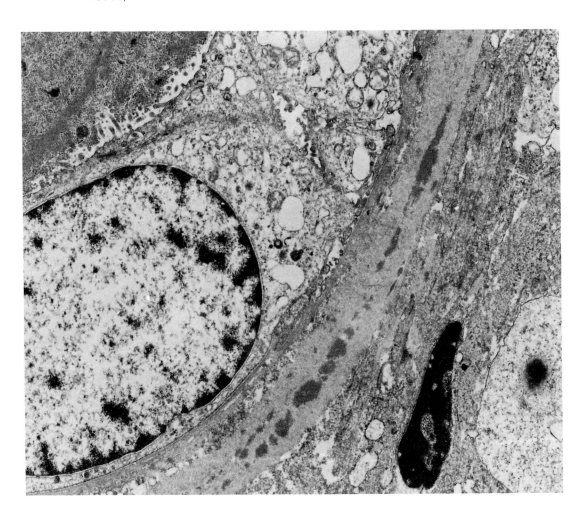

CHAPTER 7

Obstructive Uropathy and Reflux
Nephropathy

Obstructive Uropathy and Reflux Nephropathy

Obstructive Uropathy

Structural changes in the urinary tract caused by obstruction to urine outflow constitute an obstructive uropathy. Depending on the severity, site and duration of the lesion, dilatation develops proximal to the site of obstruction. In urethral obstruction, the bladder is dilated and hypertrophied and shows marked trabeculation and formation of diverticula. Back pressure on the ureter produces hydroureter, whereas back pressure on the kidney leads to hydronephrosis, with dilatation of calices and, eventually, cortical atrophy.

Clinical Features

Presenting signs and symptoms of obstructive uropathy depend on the cause, site, duration and severity of the obstruction and on whether the condition is complicated by urinary tract infection and/or renal impairment. Clinical manifestations may therefore consist of relapsing urinary tract infection, symptoms of chronic end-stage kidney failure, renal colic, prostatic symptoms and dull pain in the loins made worse by high fluid intake. In other cases, the uropathy may be discovered during an investigation undertaken to determine the cause of enlargement of the kidneys and/or bladder found on routine clinical examination. Obstructive uropathy sometimes is manifest by failure to pass a urethral catheter as a result of urethral stricture. The disease also may arise in patients with a neurologic deficit (e.g., spina bifida, paraplegia or multiple sclerosis).

The investigation of obstructive uropathy should consist of a careful history and physical examination, followed by an assessment of kidney function, particularly if the condition is bilateral. Excretion urography should be the next step; if the results of this study leave doubt as to the site of the obstruction, antigrade or retrograde pyelography may have to be undertaken.

Pathologic Changes in the Kidneys

Even in the absence of urinary tract infection, obstructive uropathy may lead to severe renal damage if left untreated. As intrapelvic pressure rises, caliceal dilatation increases and cortical atrophy develops. There may be marked interstitial fibrosis, which has been claimed to be related to extrusion of Tamm-Horsfall protein from renal tubules. The tubules often are dilated and filled with hyaline casts. The glomeruli may show hyalinization and crowding. There also may be superimposed changes relating to past or present episodes of bacterial infection with focal areas of inflammatory infiltrate in the interstitium (see Chapter

3). Obstruction and infection occurring together may also lead to papillary necrosis.

If infection develops in an obstructed kidney, hydronephrosis may be converted into pyone-phrosis. The pelvis usually is dilated and filled with pus. In advanced cases, the whole kidney may be converted into a pus-filled sac.

Vesicoureteral Reflux-Associated Nephropathy (reflux nephropathy)

This association is defined and described in Chapter 3 and encompasses renal damage associated with vesicoureteral reflux. Although bacterial infection is a major determinant of the pathologic damage induced by vesicoureteral reflux, there is evidence that when associated with high-pressure obstruction, vesicoureteral reflux may cause renal damage in the absence of infection (sterile reflux).

The severity of vesicoureteral reflux has been graded in several ways by use of cystoscopic and radiologic variables. Three grades have been recommended by the Medical Research Council (United Kingdom) Committee:

Grade I (mild): Contrast medium flows into the ureter but does not reach the kidney.

Grade II (moderate): Contrast medium flows into the ureter and reaches the kidney but does not distend the calices or ureter.

Grade III (severe): Contrast medium flows into the ureter, reaches the kidney and distends the calices, ureter, pelvis or all three. (This grade may be subdivided on the basis of degree of dilatation.)

The severity of vesicoureteral reflux is influenced by several variables, including:

(a) severity of the anatomic and functional derangement in the vesicoureteral region; this derangement tends to become less severe over time, and reflux may therefore disappear;

(b) presence of bladder outlet obstruction, unstable bladder contractions or both;

(c) vigor and efficacy of ureteral contractions;

(d) technical considerations, such as rate of contrast medium infusion, amount of contrast medium used and whether the examination is performed under general anesthesia (which is not recommended).

(e) intrarenal reflux, which represents backflow of contrast medium from the calices into the collecting tubules, a phenomenon that is occasionally seen in association with severe vesicoureteral reflux.

Two main types of vesicoureteral reflux are recognized. In focal reflux (see later), segmental corticomedullary scars are juxtaposed with dilated ("clubbed") calices.

In the generalized variety (described below), there is a variable degree of generalized dilatation of the pelvicaliceal system and ureter, associated with diffuse parenchymal "hydronephrotic" atrophy, as well as segmental scarring. Dilatation of the upper tract implies that there is an element of functional or structural urinary tract obstruction in addition to vesicoureteral reflux.

The generalized form of reflux nephropathy usually is encountered in young children with severe vesicoureteral reflux and often is bilateral. Vesicoureteral reflux may be "primary" (i.e., unassociated with another urinary tract anomaly), or there may be additional features, such as ureteral ectopia and duplication or posterior urethral valve ("secondary" reflux). In such settings, it is not unusual to find evidence of maldifferentiation (renal dysplasia) in some lobes of the kidney. It is possible that such cases represent an intrinsic anomaly of ureteral bud development of which both the ureteral abnormality resulting in vesicoureteral reflux and the renal parenchymal maldevelopment are reflections. On the other hand, intrauterine vesicoureteral reflux may cause the dysplastic renal differentiation. The changes observed in such kidneys thus represent a combination of those due to congenital maldevelopment and those due to acquired mechanisms.

The focal form of reflux nephropathy is probably always an acquired disease in the sense that the kidney has developed normally and scarring has occurred as a result of urinary tract infection in association with vesicoureteral and intrarenal reflux. The degree of impairment of renal function in patients with this form of reflux nephropathy depends on the extent of scarring, particularly in bilateral disease. Although it is apparently an acquired disease, available evidence suggests that scarring occurs during infancy or early childhood. Late deterioration in older children, adolescents and younger adults may be associated with the onset of secondary hypertension or the development of glomerular disease (focal glomerulosclerosis), which usually is identified when proteinuria is found. About 10% to 15% of patients with reflux nephropathy eventually suffer from hypertension.

It is perhaps important to stress that not all children with vesicoureteral reflux, even those who have urinary tract infection, suffer from reflux nephropathy. Failure to scar may depend on an insufficiency of micturating bladder pressure to cause intrarenal reflux, absence of renal papillae of the type associated with intrarenal reflux or lack of certain characteristics in the infecting organisms that affects their pathogenicity in the kidney. Clinical experience has shown that children who are older than about four years of age, in whom the kidneys are unscarred even though they have vesicoureteral reflux, are unlikely to have scars subsequently. Even in patients with scars, the development of new areas of scarring is an uncommon occurrence.

Reflux nephropathy usually is diagnosed in children who present with recurrent urinary tract infection. When apparently healthy schoolgirls are screened for asymptomatic bacteriuria, renal scarring is found in approximately one of every 400. In later life, reflux nephropathy may present with hypertension, particularly during pregnancy or when oral contraception is started. Renal segmental hypoplasia (the so-called Ask-Upmark kidney), which has been regarded as an important cause of hypertension in childhood and which is characterized by polar scarring and caliceal deformity, is now regarded by most authorities as a form of focal reflux nephropathy. Failure to recognize this nephropathy earlier probably stems from the selection of cases with hypertension in an age group where vesicoureteral reflux has often disappeared spontaneously and thus may no longer be demonstrable.

Obstructive Uropathy
Hydronephrosis

Fig. 7-1   Hydronephrosis due to carcinoma of ureter. Note dilated pelvis lined by thin mucosa and dilated calices. There is considerable atrophy of parenchyma.

Fig. 7-2   Hydronephrosis due to calculous obstruction. Mucosa of dilated pelvis is thickened. Calculi are seen in dilated calices.

Fig. 7-3   Hydronephrosis showing flattening of renal papillae and dilatation of collecting ducts. (hematoxylin and eosin, ×45)

Fig. 7-4   Higher magnification of Figure 7-3 showing dilated collecting ducts. (hematoxylin and eosin, ×110)

Fig. 7-5   Tubular destruction and peritubular inflammation. A large cast, probably Tamm-Horsfall protein, is seen in the tubular lumen. (periodic acid-Schiff, ×270)

Fig. 7-6   Branch of renal artery showing fragmentation of elastica. (hemotaxylin and eosin, ×110)

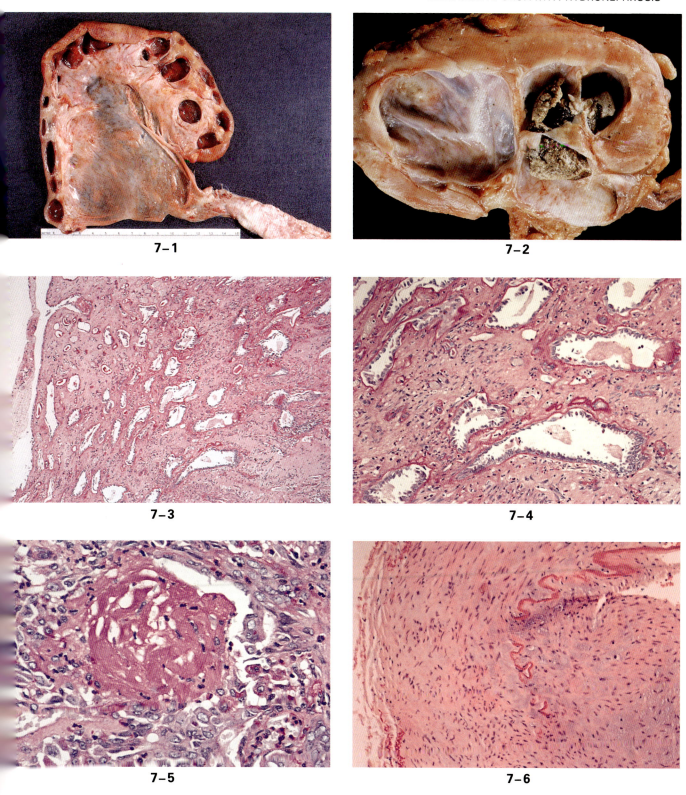

7–1

7–2

7–3

7–4

7–5

7–6

Obstructive Uropathy
Hydronephrosis

Fig. 7-7   Unilateral hydronephrosis associated with hypertension. Increased amounts of renin can be seen along a glomerular arteriole. Hypertension was cured by nephrectomy. (antirenin immunoperoxidase, ×270)

Pyonephrosis

Fig. 7-8   Pyonephrosis. Dilated renal pelvis showing mucosal inflammation and hemorrhages.

Fig. 7-9   Same case as in Figure 7-8. Purulent contents from pelvis in a bowl.

Reflux Nephropathy

Fig. 7-10   Reflux nephropathy showing large depressed scar in center with relative sparing of poles.

Fig. 7-11   Cut section of same case as in Figure 7-10 showing marked atrophy of parenchyma corresponding to the scar.

Fig. 7-12   Reflux nephropathy. Clubbed calix with overlying scar. (van Gieson's stain, ×10)

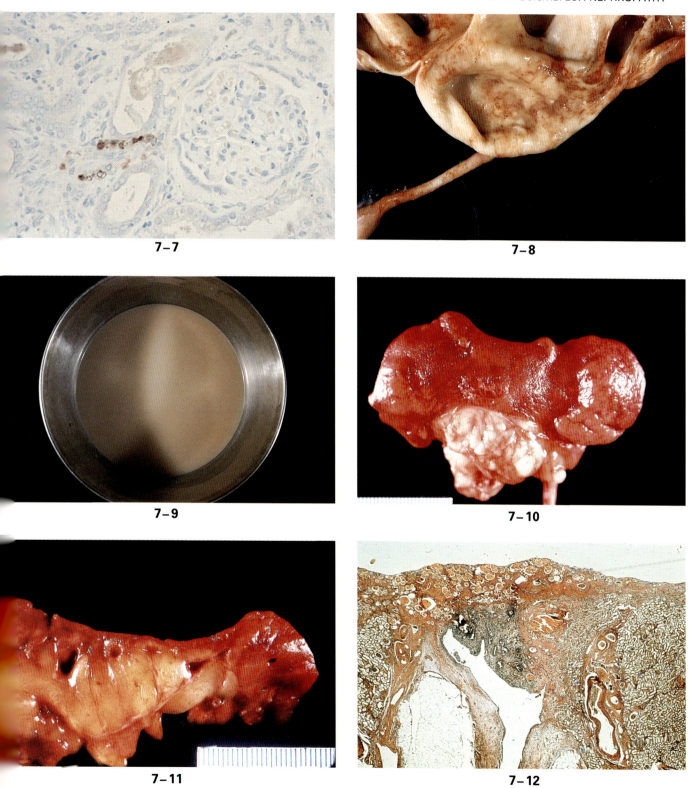

7–7

7–8

7–9

7–10

7–11

7–12

Reflux Nephropathy

Fig. 7-13 Reflux nephropathy, early stage, showing tubular atrophy and tubular dilatation as well as sclerosis of glomeruli. (periodic acid-Schiff, ×45)

Fig. 7-14 Reflux nephropathy, late stage, showing advanced atrophy, glomerular sclerosis and arteriosclerosis. (periodic acid-Schiff, ×45)

Fig. 7-15 Reflux nephropathy, advanced stage, showing almost complete disappearance of tubules and glomeruli with crowding of thick-walled blood vessels. (periodic acid-Schiff, ×100)

Fig. 7-16 Same case as in Figure 7-15. Chronic papillitis with dilatation of collecting ducts. (periodic acid-Schiff, ×45)

Fig. 7-17 Reflux nephropathy. Cast of Tamm-Horsfall protein in tubular lumen. (trichrome, ×110)

Fig. 7-18 Section sequential to section shown in Figure 7-17 stained with anti-Tamm-Horsfall antiserum. (fluorescence microscopy, ×110)

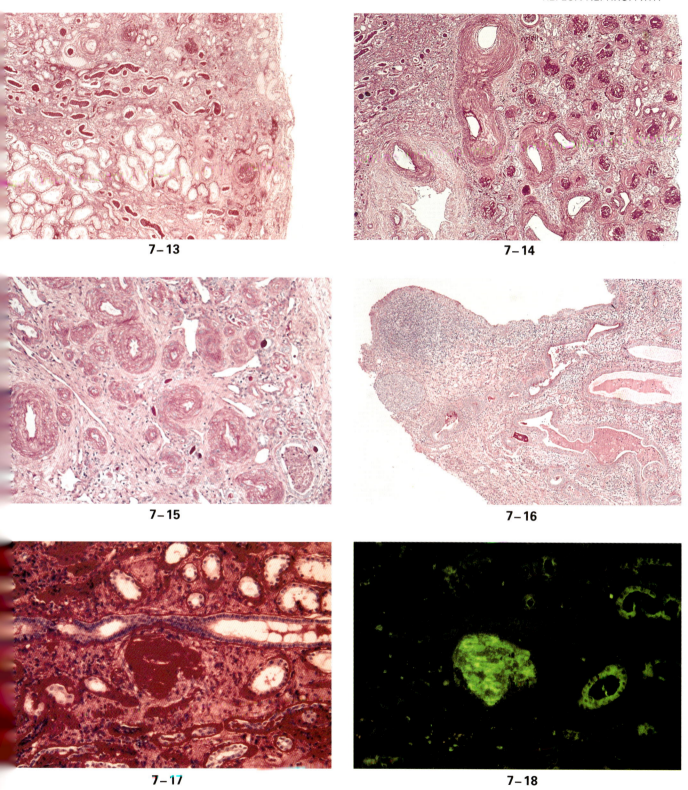

7–13

7–14

7–15

7–16

7–17

7–18

Reflux Nephropathy

Fig. 7-19 Schematic representation of grades of vesicoureteral reflux. Grade I shows normal ureteral orifice in the bladder; reflux does not reach the kidney. Grade II has a "stadium" orifice, and reflux reaches the level of the pelvis. In Grade III, the orifice is displaced laterally and has the appearance of a "golf hole"; reflux may enter the kidney (intrarenal reflux).

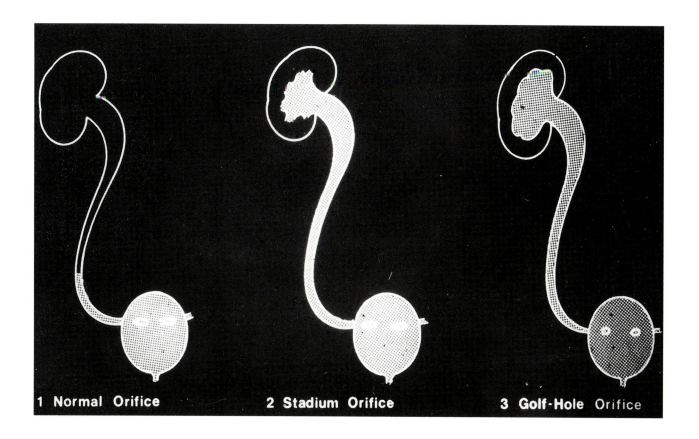

1 Normal Orifice   2 Stadium Orifice   3 Golf-Hole Orifice

Reflux Nephropathy

Fig. 7-20 Micturating cystogram in grade I vesicoureteral reflux. As bladder emp-
a to d   ties, contrast medium ascends left ureter.

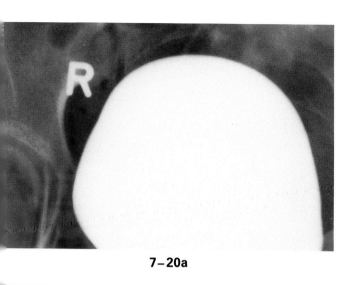

7-20a

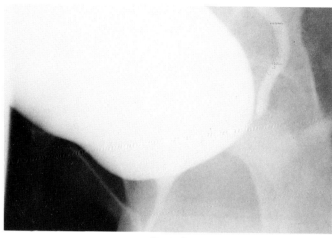
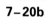

7-20b

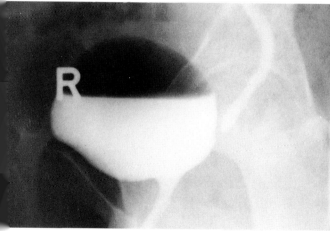

7-20c

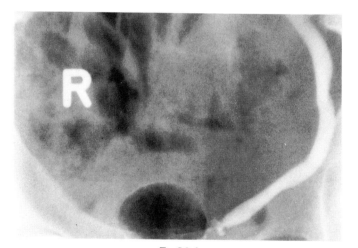

7-20d

Reflux Nephropathy

Fig. 7-21 Micturating cystogram in grade III reflux. Contrast medium has entered ureters, traveling proximally during micturition to fill both renal pelves.

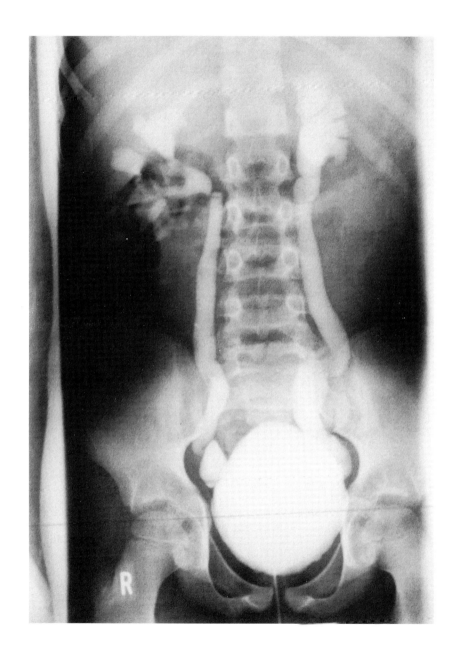

CHAPTER 8

Tubulo-interstitial Nephritis Associated with
Papillary Necrosis

Tubulo-interstitial Nephritis Associated with Papillary Necrosis

This disease is characterized by necrosis in the medulla, particularly the renal papillary structure. One or more papillae in one or both kidneys may be affected.

Papillary necrosis is associated with a number of conditions, the major ones being diabetes mellitus, obstructive uropathy, analgesic nephropathy and sickle cell disease. It also is an uncommon occurrence in newborn infants, particularly those with severe dehydration or jaundice, and is seen on rare occasions after retrograde pyelography. Pyelonephritis may complicate each of these conditions. Hematuria, pain in the flank or abdomen, chills and fever are the most common symptoms. Acute renal failure with oliguria or anemia may occur. Sloughing of papillae occurs without symptoms in rare instances in patients with chronic urinary tract infection, and the necrotic tissue may be passed in the urine.

Diabetes Mellitus

Papillary necrosis frequently is associated with diabetes mellitus. The pathogenetic mechanism responsible for the papillary damage is not clear; however, the damage may be due to reduction of blood supply and/or infection, which occurs with an increased incidence or severity in diabetes mellitus.

Obstructive Uropathy

Papillary necrosis is associated with obstruction to the outflow of urine below the renal pelvis. The pathogenetic mechanism that causes the renal damage is not known, although infection and impairment of papillary blood supply due to ureteral obstruction may be responsible.

Analgesic Nephropathy (see also Chapter 5)

The gross and microscopic features of analgesic nephropathy differ and often can be differentiated from those seen in papillary necrosis associated with diabetes mellitus or obstructive uropathy (see Chapter 5 and Table IV).

Macroscopic Findings: In diabetes mellitus and obstructive uropathy, usually but not always, both kidneys are affected. An affected kidney may be enlarged or normal but is sometimes smaller than normal. The subcapsular surface may show small white abscesses. Necrotic areas in the papillae may vary in size and shape and have congested borders. When necrotic papillae slough, they leave a ragged surface. In old necrotic papillae, foci of calcification may occur. In obstructive forms, the renal pelvis is dilated and manifests the features of obstructive uropathy (see Chapter 7).

Microscopic Findings: Medullary areas of necrosis are devoid of cells, and necrotic tubules appear as empty spaces. Such tubules may contain nuclear debris and bacteria in their lumina. In the border between necrotic and viable tissue, there

Table IV Differential Diagnosis of Papillary Necrosis in Diabetes Mellitus and Analgesic Nephropathy

Acute (diabetes mellitus)	Chronic (analgesics)
Unilateral or bilateral	Always bilateral
Several papillae affected	Almost all papillae affected
All necroses at the same stage	Different stages of necrosis
Yellow	Brown
Zone of demarcation with wall of polymorphonuclear leukocytes	Zone of demarcation without inflammatory reaction
No cystic change at zone of demarcation	Cystlike cavities at zone of demarcation
Calcification: rare	Calcification: frequent
Clinical course: acute, severe illness	Clinical course: protracted, relapsing
Prognosis: poor	Prognosis: much better than in acute type

is a zone of polymorphonuclear neutrophils. An eosinophilic deposit may be present in the interstitial tissue. Later, epithelium grows over the surface of a sloughed papilla. In the nonnecrotic medulla, there may be evidence of acute bacterial tubulo-interstitial nephritis. The cortex may show tubular loss and atrophy, with interstitial fibrosis and chronic inflammatory cell infiltration. In such areas, the glomeruli may be sclerotic. The glomeruli also may show the various lesions associated with diabetes mellitus (see volume on glomerular diseases). Radiologic abnormalities in papillary necrosis have been described (see analgesic nephropathy, Chapter 5).

Hemorrhagic Necrosis of Papillae in the Newborn

Renal hemorrhage is sometimes seen in newborn infants, particularly premature infants, as part of generalized bleeding. Hemorrhagic infarction of the kidneys may be associated with renal vein thrombosis in infants with severe diarrheal disease and marked dehydration. However, hemorrhagic necrosis of renal papillae may occur in the neonatal period unassociated with renal vein thrombosis. The cause of the lesion is obscure, and there usually is fetal anoxia, during the intra-uterine or neonatal period as a result of prolonged labor or intra-uterine asphyxia. The mechanism may be related to a neurovascular disturbance that results in shunting of blood, bypassing the cortex and leading to cortical ischemia and medullary hyperemia.

Macroscopic Findings: Both kidneys are larger than normal. The medulla is deeply hemorrhagic, but the cortex appears normal. Hemorrhage is sharply circumscribed and limited to the renal pyramids in most areas, with gross destruction of the medulla. No thrombi are found in renal veins or the inferior vena cava.

Microscopic Findings: There is diffuse hemorrhage in the renal pyramids. Masses of red cells in the interstitium separate and compress the tubules. In many areas, the tubular epithelial cells show varying stages of degeneration and necrosis.

Tubulo-interstitial Nephritis Associated with Papillary Necrosis
Diabetes Mellitus

Fig. 8-1 Necrosis of tip of papilla.

Fig. 8-2 Histologic section of necrotic papilla shown in Figure 8-1. Coagulation necrosis and small hemorrhagic area in tip. (hematoxylin and eosin, ×45)

Fig. 8-3 Severe and extensive papillary necrosis. Necrotic papillae are yellow and friable and are surrounded by a zone of congestion.

Fig. 8-4 Section from necrotic papilla show disintegration of papillary tissue and scattered inflammatory cells. (hematoxylin and eosin, ×270)

Sickle Cell Disease

Fig. 8-5 Nephrectomy for massive hemorrhage in a patient with sickle cell trait. Blood in tip of papilla (upper right) and small blood clot in corresponding calix.

Fig. 8-6 Section of papilla shown in Figure 8-5. Large capillary aneurysms are seen under the mucosa, which is partly sloughed off. (hematoxylin and eosin, ×40)

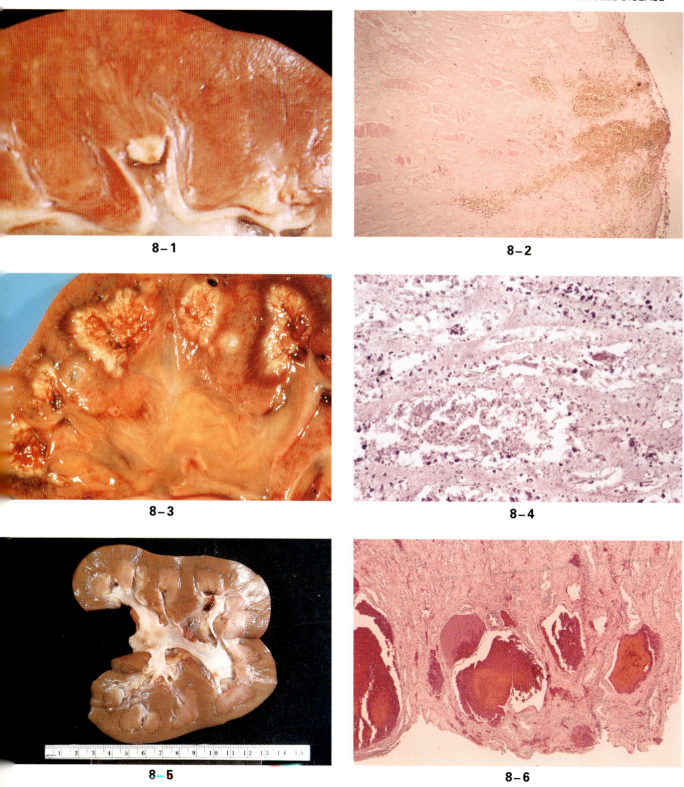

8–1

8–2

8–3

8–4

8–5

8–6

Hemorrhagic Necrosis of Papillae in Newborn

Fig. 8-7 Extensive hemorrhagic necrosis of renal papillae in a dehydrated newborn infant.

Fig. 8-8 Same specimen as in Figure 8-7 after formaldehyde fixation.

Fig. 8-9 Histologic section of specimen shown in Figure 8-8. Massive hemorrhage in papilla and medulla. (hematoxylin and eosin, ×10)

Papillary Necrosis Associated with Vascular Disease

Fig. 8-10 Necrotizing papillitis in a case of arterionephrosclerosis showing necrosis and inflammation at tip. (periodic acid-Schiff, ×270)

Fig. 8-11 Advanced scleroderma and candidal sepsis. Papillary necrosis and hemorrhage (arrowhead).

Fig. 8-12 Same case as in Figure 8-11. Section of papilla and of adjacent inner medulla showing bland necrosis. (hematoxylin and eosin, ×45)

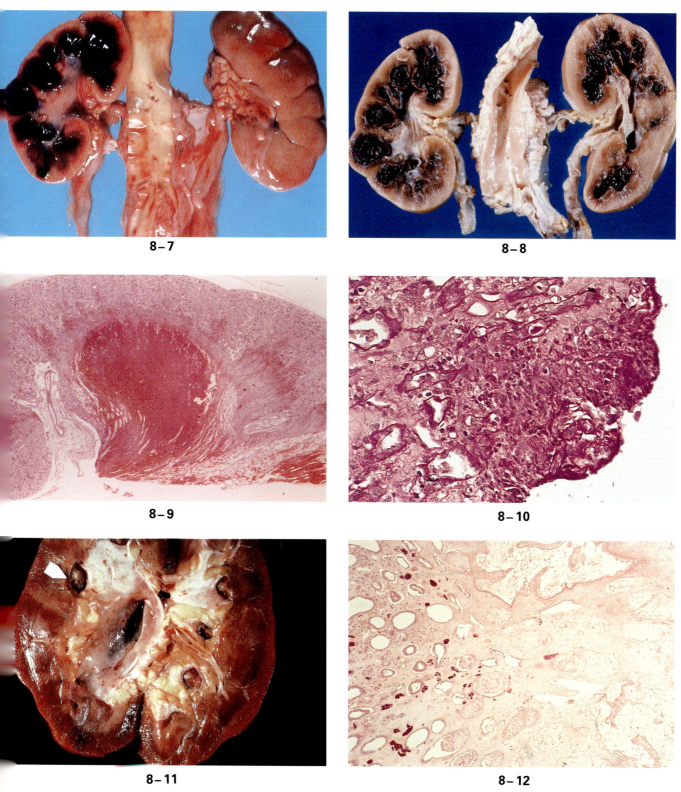

8–7

8–8

8–9

8–10

8–11

8–12

Papillary Necrosis Associated with Vascular Disease

Fig. 8-13 Same case as in Figure 8-12. Another necrotic papilla showing fragmentation of necrotic tissue. (hematoxylin and eosin, ×45)

Fig. 8-14 Necrotic fragmented tissue permeated by fungal hyphae. (periodic acid-Schiff, ×430)

Fig. 8-15 Papillary necrosis in an elderly man with secondary amyloidosis. Amyloid deposits were found almost exclusively in walls of blood vessels and in interstitial tissue of medulla and papilla. Necrotic papilla are separated from medulla (right side of picture). (hematoxylin and eosin, ×3)

Fig. 8-16 Same section as in Figure 8-15. Necrotic papilla at point of separation from medulla showing leukocytic infiltration. (hematoxylin and eosin, ×270)

Fig. 8-17 Same case as in Figure 8-16. Necrotic papilla showing pink deposits of amyloid. (Congo red, ×45)

Fig. 8-18 Same section as in Figure 8-17, under polarized light. Amyloid deposits show dichroic staining (red and green). (Congo red, ×270)

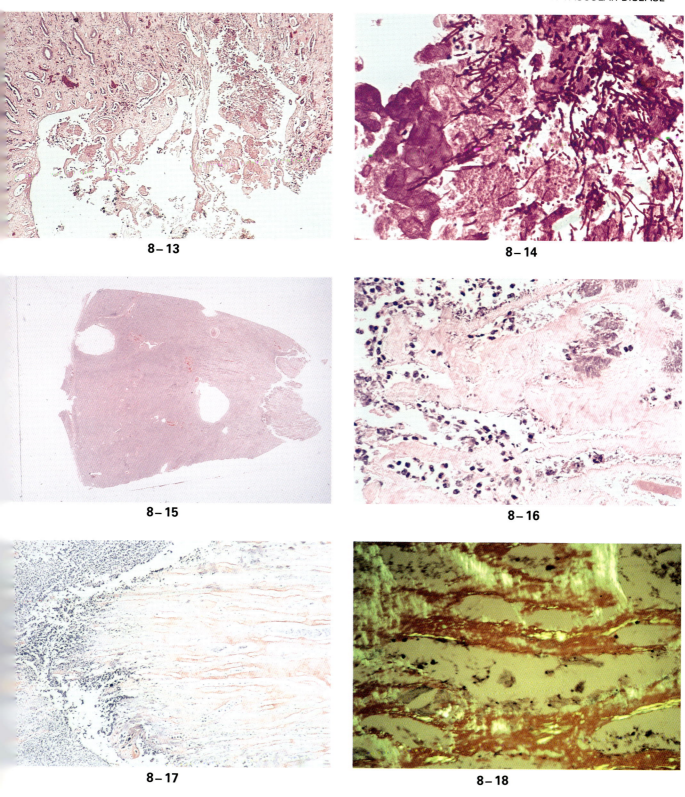

8–13

8–14

8–15

8–16

8–17

8–18

Papillary Necrosis

Fig. 8-19 Sickle cell disease. Excretory urogram of right kidney in a 22-year-old woman with painless hematuria. Loss of cupping of calix (arrow) with irregular extension of contrast medium into region of pyramid.

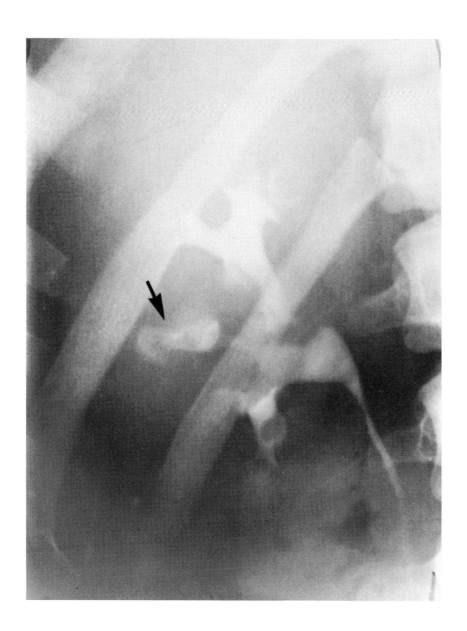

CHAPTER 9

Heavy Metal-Induced Tubular and Tubulo-interstitial Lesions

Heavy Metal-Induced Tubular and Tubulo-interstitial Lesions

Lead Nephropathy

When renal lesions are caused by acute or chronic lead intoxication, the disease is known as lead nephropathy.

In cases of acute intoxication, two to four days after ingestion of lead (e.g., lead-containing paint), patients suffer from hypersalivation, vomiting, abdominal colic, constipation, proteinuria and anuria. Urinary excretion of lead (2 to 18 mg/24 hours) is transient.

Patients with chronic plumbism (e.g., from prolonged industrial exposure to lead) show generalized weakness, anorexia, fatigue, tremor, headache, constipation and muscle weakness. Several years after the onset of symptoms, hypertension may develop. Urinary excretion of lead is increased (1.2 to 1.8 mg/24 hours), but sometimes only after administration of EDTA (ethylenediamine tetraacetate).

Light and Electron Microscopic Findings: In the acute or subacute form, epithelial cells of the cortical tubules, particularly the proximal ones and those of the loops of Henle, show nuclear inclusion bodies. Such bodies are mostly round, 2 to 7 μm in diameter and sometimes are surrounded by a clear halo. They stain moderately with eosin, are positive with periodic acid-Schiff and Ziehl-Neelsen, stain red with Giemsa and toluidine blue,

Masson's trichrome and Mallory's stain, are positive with Luxol fast blue and are negative with Sudan red and the Feulgen method. With Goldner's trichrome, the center of the inclusion body stains green, whereas the rim stains red. By autoradiography (210 Pb) in experimental lead intoxication, traces of lead can be found embedded in the proteinaceous matrix of the inclusion bodies.

As can also be shown in experimental lead intoxication, the tubules may exhibit necrosis and pathologic mitoses of the epithelial cells as well as cystic dilatation and basophilic or oncocytic hyperplasia. Adenomas and carcinomas also have been observed.

Electron microscopy reveals that the nuclear inclusion bodies have compact cores and outer zones consisting of a meshwork of fibrils. (Bismuth inclusion bodies, which are now rarely seen because bismuth is no longer used in the management of syphilis, can be differentiated from lead inclusion bodies because the former have homogeneous structure.)

Although patients with chronic plumbism may suffer from chronic renal insufficiency as a result of tubulo-interstitial nephritis, the relationship between the two entities and the possible pathogenesis of chronic renal injury in such patients are unclear. Chronic lead intoxication is manifested by chronic tubulo-interstitial disease with interstitial fibrosis as well as by arteriosclerosis. The histologic picture may be difficult to distinguish from that seen in the common form of nephrosclerosis because lead inclusion bodies usually are absent. Progression to renal failure has been reported.

Mercury Nephropathy

Mercury nephropathy may serve as a prototype of renal damage induced by many heavy metals. It consists of acute tubular injury as well as chronic tubulo-interstitial nephritis, depending on the dosage and duration of exposure.

Acute intoxication usually is caused by accidental or suicidal ingestion of inorganic mercurial compounds or by industrial exposure. Ingestion causes severe gastrointestinal symptoms, including nausea, vomiting, abdominal pain and diarrhea. This symptom complex is followed by circulatory collapse and oliguria or anuria. If urine is examined before the onset of anuria, it is found to contain protein, red cells, excess glucose and amino acids. Mortality with large doses exceeds 50%.

Macroscopic examination shows that the kidneys are enlarged, swollen and pale. Microscopic studies demonstrate changes that are especially striking in the middle and terminal (straight) segments of the proximal tubules. The changes consist of granular or vacuolar degeneration of the cytoplasm, together with nuclear pyknosis and karyolysis. There is rapid progression to necrosis and desquamation of cells as well as accumulation of debris in the lumina. Early calcification of necrotic cells is seen frequently. Electron microscopy demonstrates loss of brush borders and mitochondrial changes, including swelling, pyknosis and fragmentation.

Regeneration begins after three to five days and is accompanied by clearing of debris from the lumina, first of the proximal and then of the distal tubules. Injured tubules are dilated and lined by flat basophilic cells, which often show mitoses. The cells soon become cuboidal or low columnar and gradually develop brush borders, mitochondria and endoplasmic reticulum and assume their normal configuration. Interstitial edema and inflammation may persist for some time.

Chronic intoxication is due mainly to industrial exposure in such occupations as manufacture of scientific instruments or mercury vapor lamps or in occupations in which infectants or pesticides are commonly used. In some cases, long-term application to the skin of ointments that contain mercury compounds leads to mercury nephropathy. In mild cases, slight to moderate proteinuria may be the only manifestation. With more severe damage, there may be nephrotic syndrome or Fanconi's syndrome with proximal renal tubular acidosis. Renal insufficiency is a frequent occurrence and may lead to renal failure.

On microscopic examination, the glomeruli appear to be preserved, although patients with nephrotic syndrome usually show membranous glomerulonephritis. In the earlier stages, some proximal tubules are lined by nearly normal cells, but many show very flat epithelium. Tubular lumina are dilated and often are filled with cellular debris. Interstitial tissue is edematous and contains a sparse distribution of inflammatory cells, mostly lymphocytes. With progression of damage, the tubules are gradually obliterated by fibrosis and inflammatory, mainly lymphocytic, infiltrate. Tubules that remain are dilated and lined by cuboidal or flat epithelium. The lumina usually are empty.

Cisplatin Nephropathy

Cisplatin (cis-dichlorodiammine platinum II) is an effective anticancer drug that causes renal damage; the damage is similar to that produced by other heavy metals. Acute renal failure, which is prob-

119

ably due to tubular degeneration or necrosis, is common, but with the usual therapeutic dosages and proper hydration, it usually is mild. However, despite the mildness of the acute renal failure, it may progress to chronic failure. The latter may also develop insidiously. Severe tubular damage with interstitial fibrosis and inflammation as well as microcystic tubular dilatation is found in laboratory animals given repeated doses of cisplatin.

Chronic renal injury in human beings is manifested by tubular atrophy and interstitial disease. Tubules become moderately dilated, are lined by cuboidal or flattened cells and sometimes contain debris in their lumina. Some cells show vacuoles and, occasionally, pyknotic nuclei. Interstitial tissue shows considerable edema and fibrosis, with separation of tubules. There are small collections of inflammatory cells, mainly lymphocytes and histiocytes, and calcium deposits in rare instances.

With progression of damage, tubular atrophy becomes more pronounced. The tubules are considerably, although irregularly, dilated, and the lining cells are flat. Calcified cells and calcified cellular casts, occasional hyaline casts and even polymorphonuclear casts are seen in the lumina. There is considerable interstitial fibrosis and fairly numerous cellular infiltrates of lymphocytes, histiocytes, plasma cells and some polymorphonuclear leukocytes.

The glomeruli are at first preserved but later may develop mesangial widening and sclerosis. Nephrotic syndrome has not been reported, but moderate proteinuria may be present.

Cadmium Nephropathy

Clinical Features: After inhalation of cadmium fumes (e.g., by workers in cadmium industries or welders who use cadmium-containing alloys), acute respiratory symptoms or pulmonary edema may develop apart from irritation of the nasopharynx. In chronic intoxication, the most important renal symptom is proteinuria. Unlike the glomerular and tubular proteinuria usually encountered, the excreted protein has a relatively low molecular weight of 20,000 to 30,000. It consists mainly of small globulins, including β_2-microglobulin and immunoglobulin light chains. The urinary protein does not show the same reactions to routine laboratory tests as it does in cases with glomerular lesions. Tubular damage also is manifested by aminoaciduria, renal glycosuria and impairment of ability to concentrate the urine. There is no documented proof of progression to renal insufficiency.

Light and Electron Microscopic Findings: Light microscopy demonstrates no distinctive change, even in relation to the low-molecular-weight (tubular?) proteinuria. Electron microscopic studies in laboratory animals have shown swelling of mitochondria in tubular cells and an increase in the number of lysosomes in the proximal tubules. Tubular reabsorption of protein appears to be intact.

Other Heavy Metal-Induced Nephropathies

Gold Nephropathy

Organic compounds of gold are used in the management of rheumatoid arthritis. Renal injury develops gradually with such manifestations as proteinuria, microhematuria, nephrotic syndrome and chronic renal failure. Occasionally, acute renal failure occurs, with severe tubular damage and inclusions of gold in the cell cytoplasm. The latter is best demonstrated by microprobe analysis. In patients with nephrotic syndrome, gold has been found in the tubules but not in the glomeruli. The mechanism of action of gold and other heavy metals (mercury, iron) in the causation of nephrotic syndrome has not been established.

Silver Nephropathy

Chronic ingestion of silver salts (used in the past for the management of peptic ulcer) causes deposition of silver in glomerular basement membranes and basement membranes of the interstitial capillaries but no clinical manifestations. Intraperitoneal injection of silver compounds into laboratory animals leads to tubular degeneration and interstitial deposition of silver.

Copper Nephropathy

Copper sulfate can cause acute renal failure associated with tubular degeneration, especially in the ascending limb of the loops of Henle and in the distal convoluted tubules. In chronic intoxication, proximal tubules show cellular degeneration, desquamation and fragmentation, with coarse granular casts in their lumina. Many proximal tubular lining cells contain fine granules of copper that stain blue with hematoxylin, purple with periodic acid-Schiff and black with rubeanic acid.

Iron Nephropathy

Iron may cause renal damage (tubular necrosis and acute renal failure) when ingested in large doses in its sulfate form. Organic iron compounds have been shown to induce nephrotic syndrome in laboratory animals.

Hemolysis of any type often leads to deposition of iron (hemosiderin) in the tubular cells (hemolytic anemia, sickle cell disease, hemoglobinuria, aortic valve prosthesis, hemochromatosis, hemosiderosis).

Heavy Metal-Induced Tubulo-interstitial Nephritis
Lead Nephropathy

Fig. 9-1   Lead nephropathy. Proximal tubular cells contain red-staining ("lipofuscin") granules in the cytoplasm and show slight thickening of tubular basement membranes. (periodic acid-Schiff, ×1100)

Fig. 9-2   Tubular epithelial cells showing typical intranuclear eosinophilic inclusion bodies. (hematoxylin and eosin, ×1700)

Fig. 9-3   Lead Nephropathy, chronic. Tubular atrophy, interstitial fibrosis and arteriosclerosis. (periodic acid-Schiff, ×430)

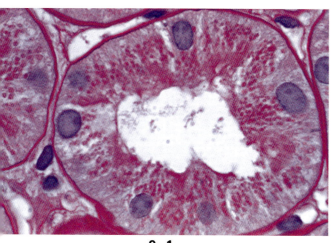

9–1

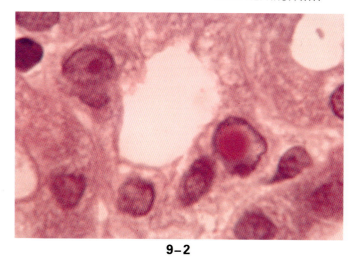

9–2

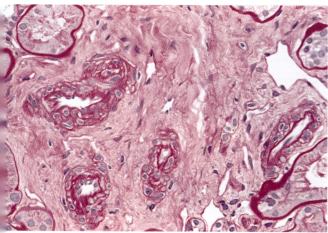

9–3

Mercury

Fig. 9-4 Mercury poisoning, acute. Almost complete necrosis of proximal convoluted tubules. (hematoxylin and eosin, ×135)

Fig. 9-5 Mercury poisoning, chronic. Cut surface of kidney showing swollen, mottled, reddish and yellowish parenchyma.

Fig. 9-6 Mercury poisoning, chronic. Tubular degeneration and interstitial edema and fibrosis. Dilated tubules are lined by flattened cells. Desquamated cells and granular material are seen in lumina. (hematoxylin and eosin, ×110)

Fig. 9-7 Mercury poisoning, chronic. Another case showing more advanced lesions, including tubular atrophy, interstitial fibrosis and chronic inflammation. (hematoxylin and eosin, ×270)

Fig. 9-8 Same case as in Figure 9-7. Microprobe spectrum of dense body shown in Figure 9-19. Spectrum shows two yellow peaks characteristic of mercury. (Red peaks represent osmium from fixative, and nickel and copper from grid and specimen holder.)

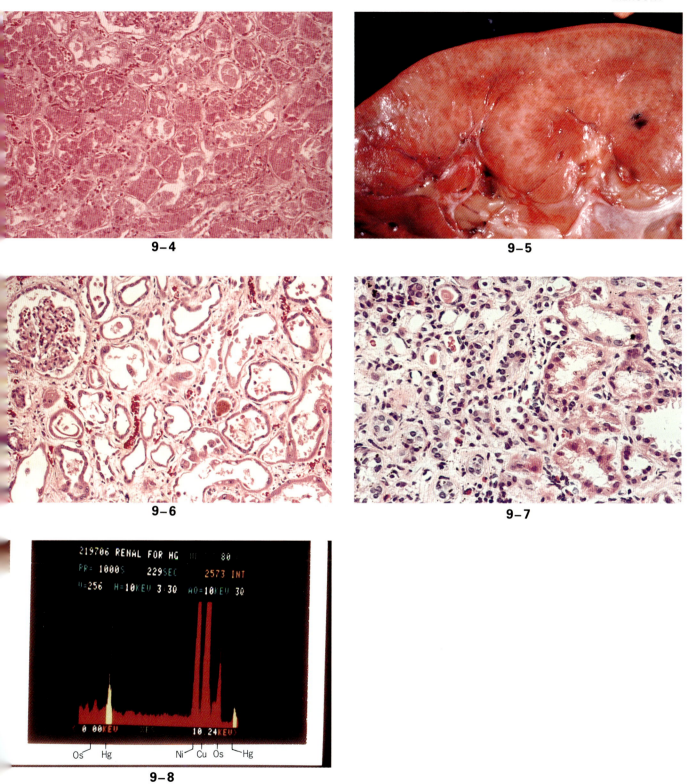

9–4

9–5

9–6

9–7

9–8

Cisplatin

Fig. 9-9   Cisplatin poisoning, chronic, in a patient treated for a malignant tumor. Tubules showing degeneration and flattening of epithelial cells. Interstitial edema, fibrosis and focal inflammation also are seen. (hematoxylin and eosin, ×270)

Fig. 9-10   Cisplatin poisoning. Biopsy specimen from same case as in Figure 9-9, six months later. Progression of tubular atrophy and interstitial fibrosis. Desquamated calcified epithelium is seen in one part of lumen. Patient showed moderate proteinuria and renal insufficiency. (hematoxylin and eosin, ×270)

Copper

Fig. 9-11   Copper poisoning, chronic. Swelling, degeneration and desquamation of proximal tubular epithelial cells. (hematoxylin and eosin, ×430)

Fig. 9-12   Copper poisoning, chronic. Same case as in Figure 9-11. Cytoplasm of tubular cells contains granules of copper that stain purplish. (periodic acid-Schiff, ×430)

Fig. 9-13   Copper poisoning, chronic. Section from the case shown in Figure 9-12, stained for copper. Copper granules appear greenish black. (rubeanic acid, ×430)

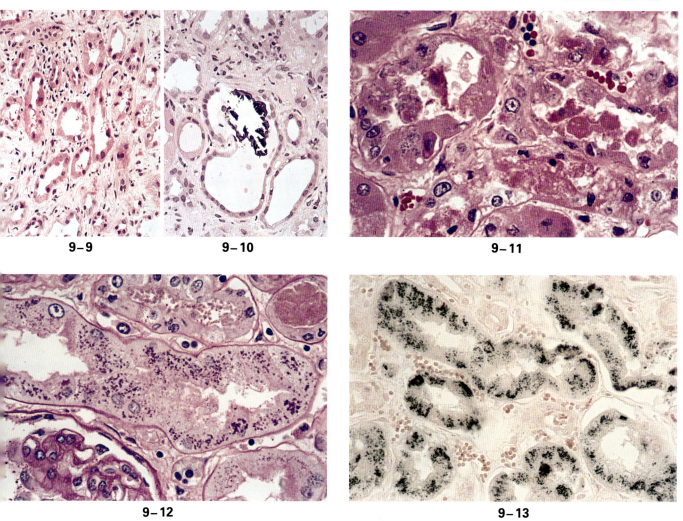

9−9　　　　　　　　9−10　　　　　　　　　　　　9−11

9−12　　　　　　　　　　　　　　　　9−13

Lead Nephropathy

Fig. 9-14 Lead nephropathy. Same case as in Figure 9-1. Proximal tubular cells showing large lysosomes containing granules of osmiophilic material. (electron micrograph, ×22,000)

Fig. 9-15 Proximal tubular epithelial cell showing a dense intranuclear inclusion body near center of nucleus. Next to it is a typical nucleolus. (electron micrograph, ×6000)

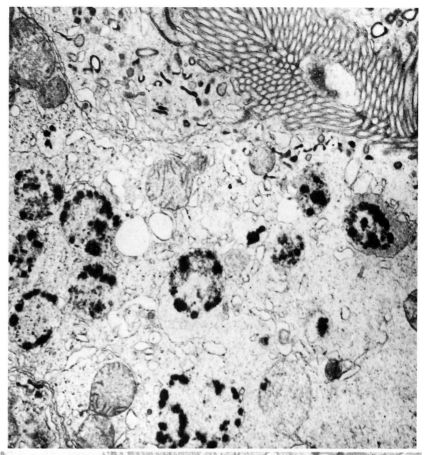
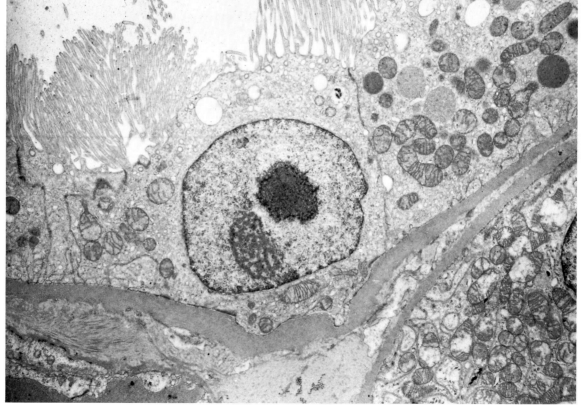

Lead Nephropathy

Fig. 9-16 High magnification of intranuclear inclusion body in another case of lead nephropathy. Inclusion body consists of fine fibrillar material at periphery and more compact material in center. (electron micrograph, × 55,000)

Fig. 9-17 Bismuth inclusion body (for comparison with lead inclusion body). Bismuth inclusion body is round and homogeneously dense in osmium-fixed tissue. (Stippling may be noted with formalin fixation.) Smaller, dense bismuth inclusion bodies also are present in mitochondria. (electron micrograph, × 12,000)

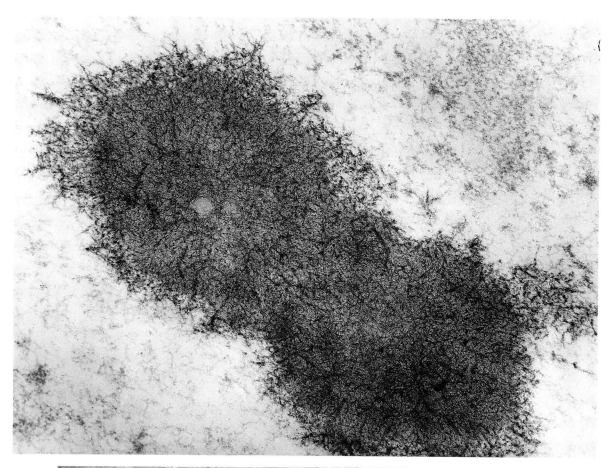

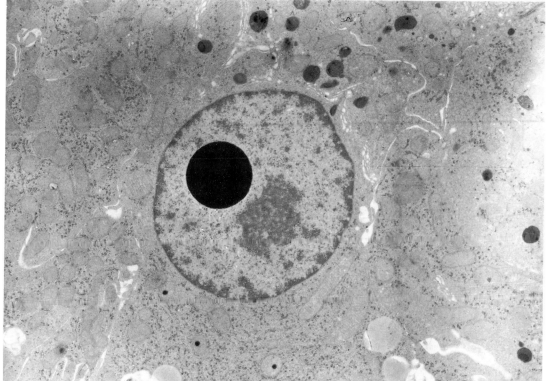

Mercury

Fig. 9-18 Mercury poisoning, chronic. Same case as in Figure 9-7 (tissue reprocessed from paraffin block). Proximal tubular cells appear vocuolated. One cell contains a small dense body in a cytoplasm (arrow). (electron micrograph, ×15,000)

Fig. 9-19 Same case as in Figure 9-18. Higher magnification of a similar dense body. (electron micrograph, ×75,000)

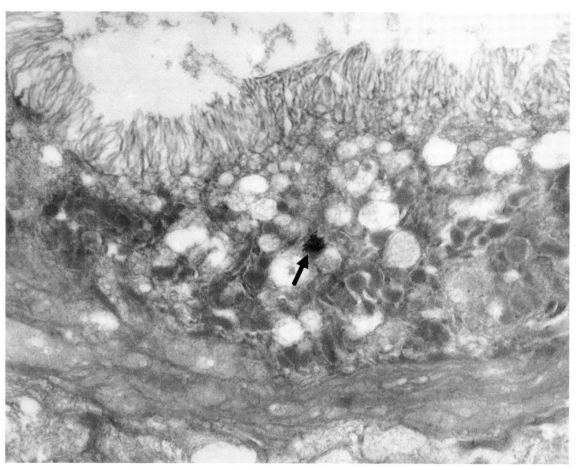
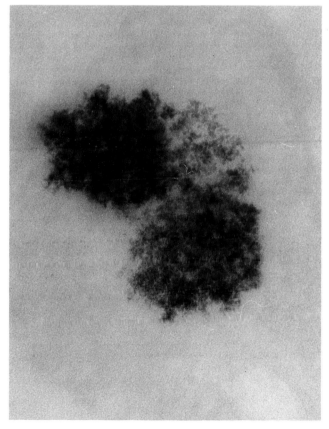

Silver

Fig. 9-20 Silver poisoning, chronic. Long-term administration of silver nitrate to a rat. Granules of silver are seen in glomerular basement membranes. (electron micrograph, ×17,000)

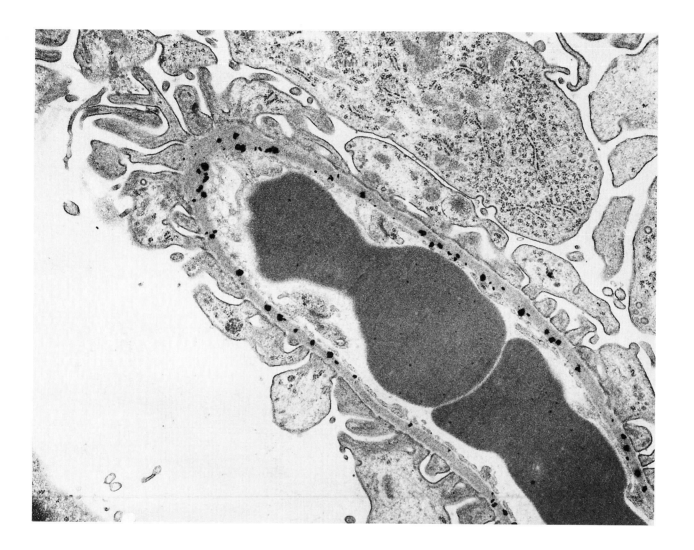

CHAPTER 10

Acute Tubular Injury/Necrosis

Acute Tubular Injury/Necrosis

Acute renal failure is a clinical term that refers to abrupt suppression of excretory renal function. It is characterized by a decrease in the 24-hour volume of urine and by accumulation of waste products in the blood (uremia). Causes of acute renal failure usually are classified under one of three headings: prerenal, postrenal or renal. Prerenal causes include hypovolemia resulting from hemorrhage, fluid loss or sequestration (diarrhea, vomiting, extensive burns, peritonitis, massive edema), cardiovascular failure (myocardial infarction, sepsis) and in rare instances, transient hypotension.

Postrenal causes relate to obstruction along the urinary tract.

Renal causes include such entities as acute glomerulonephritis, necrotizing arteritis, malignant hypertension, acute interstitial nephritis and papillary necrosis. The most frequent cause, and therefore the most important cause in the clinical setting, is the tubular damage called "acute tubular necrosis." This necrosis accounts for perhaps 75% of all cases of acute renal failure and carries considerable mortality.

Acute tubular necrosis may be divided into two categories: toxic and ischemic. The toxic form is due to nephrotoxins (heavy metals, solvents, drugs) and is manifested by obvious necrosis of tubular cells.

In the ischemic form, cellular injury is more subtle and is presumed to be due to decreased perfusion ("vasomotor nephropathy"). Nephrotoxic damage is dealt with elsewhere in this book but will be discussed here in greater detail. Special attention will be devoted to acute tubular necrosis due to vasomotor nephropathy.

Renal ischemia, other than that caused by vascular obstruction, is initiated, in most cases, by the same processes that induce prerenal failure (see above). Even a brief episode of hypotension (e.g., fainting spell) may lead, on occasion, to vasomotor nephropathy. Severe hypotension secondary to a severe crushing injury, shock or septic abortion, for example, often induces severe renal ischemia. The major difference between prerenal failure and acute tubular necrosis is that the former can be promptly reversed by appropriate measures (volume repletion, improvement of cardiac action), whereas the latter is unaffected by these measures. It follows that differentiation between these two conditions is important therapeutically and prognostically.

Certain data derived from urinalysis may provide helpful clues for differentiation. Urine volume is reduced in both conditions, usually to less than 400 ml/24 hours, although in some (20% to 30%) cases, the failure in acute tubular necrosis is nonoliguric, with urine volume approaching normal but with rising blood urea nitrogen and creatinine levels. The presence or absence of proteinuria is not a helpful sign. Hematuria, particularly when it is accompanied by red cell casts, is an indication of glomerular disease, whereas leukocyturia points to acute pyelonephritis or papillary necrosis. A small or moderate number of hyaline and finely granular casts is seen in prerenal failure; in acute tubular necrosis, there are many granular casts (which often exhibit a brownish tinge), epithelial cells and epithelial cell casts. Urine specific gravity and osmolality are the same as for blood plasma (isosthenuria) in acute tubular necrosis but are high in prerenal failure. Urinary sodium concentration is high in acute tubular necrosis but is low or normal in prerenal failure.

The appearance of an affected kidney depends on the severity of the insult and on elapsed time. In earlier stages, the kidney is enlarged and swollen, the cortex is pale and the medulla is congested and dark, but later the appearance is more varied.

Nephrotoxic Acute Tubular Necrosis (see also Chapter 5)

Microscopic examination demonstrates that the classic changes of nephrotoxic acute tubular necrosis are exemplified by heavy metal poisoning, such as that caused by mercury. Mercury salts cause extensive degeneration and necrosis of the epithelium of proximal tubules, which is particularly prominent in the straight segments of all or most of the nephrons. Similar changes are observed with uranyl, bismuth, arsenic, cisplatin and, on occasion, many other heavy metals (see Chapter 9). A gaseous arsenic compound, arsine (AsH_3), causes direct tubular damage and also induces hemolysis and hemoglobinuria, which contribute to the renal failure.

Solvents such as carbon tetrachloride are probably responsible for more cases of nephrotoxic acute tubular necrosis than are heavy metals. This condition commonly develops in persons who use such solvents for cleaning purposes in poorly ventilated spaces. Alcoholics appear to be particularly susceptible. The cause of death is more often extrarenal, due to damage to the liver or central nervous system.

Glycols (ethylene glycol, diethylene glycol, dioxane) produce "vacuolar" degeneration in the proximal convoluted tubules, which is characterized by formation of large vacuoles, progressive disruption of cytoplasm, necrosis, shedding of cells and, in many cases, precipitation of oxalate crystals in the lumina. In severe cases, there may be extensive cortical necrosis. Ethylene glycol is used as automotive antifreeze and sometimes is imbibed by alcoholics. As with carbon tetrachloride, the cause of death is often extrarenal, due to central nervous system depression, liver failure or cardiac failure.

In the clinical setting, the most common cause of nephrotoxic acute tubular necrosis is administration of therapeutic agents, such as antibiotics (aminoglycosides, cephalosporins), nonsteroidal antiinflammatory drugs and mercurial diuretics (see Table II, p. 59). The severity of the various clinical manifestations, such as proteinuria, cylindruria, hypernatremia and, most importantly, deterioration of renal function, varies with the drug, dosage and duration of therapy, state of hydration and preexisting or concomitant renal disease of other origin. Discontinuation of therapy usually leads to clearing of symptoms, but severe damage, particularly after prolonged drug administration, may progress to the typical syndrome of nephrotoxic renal failure. Histologic changes in mild cases are limited to "cloudy swelling" and vacuolation of proximal tubular cells, but in more severe cases, progression to necrosis is observed.

On occasion, iodinated radiographic contrast media cause urinary abnormalities and renal insufficiency by a variety of mechanisms, such as reduction of renal blood flow, intrarenal osmotic effect and direct tubule toxicity, which may be severe. Dehydration is a contributing factor, and diabetics appear to be more prone to renal failure.

Poorly soluble sulfonamides are no longer used in therapy because of their tendency to precipitate in the kidneys, blocking the distal tubules and causing degeneration and necrosis of the epithelial lining. Clinical findings include hematuria, pyuria and crystalluria, as well as pain and, occasionally, renal colic and renal insufficiency. Sulfonamides also may cause a hypersensitivity reaction in the form of acute interstitial nephritis and even generalized necrotizing arteritis.

Ischemic Acute Tubular Necrosis (acute vasomotor nephropathy)

In ischemic acute tubular necrosis, changes in the proximal tubules are more subtle and are easily obscured by postmortem autolysis. In biopsy material, cellular degeneration and necrosis are almost always present but involve only single cells or small scattered patches, and these changes lead to shedding of cell fragments and whole cells into the lumen, with denudation of segments of the basement membranes. Such focal necrotic lesions also occur in the distal tubules. With more severe damage, there is focal fragmentation of the basement membranes ("tubulorrhexis"), infiltration of tubules by inflammatory cells and, sometimes, escape of tubular contents into the interstitium. Such casts may protrude into small veins, elevating the endothelium. Tubulorrhexis is a more obvious, but less specific, lesion; it also is seen in glomerulonephritis and is particularly prominent in acute interstitial nephritis.

Many tubules are dilated and are lined by flattened epithelium, partly because of shedding of the cytoplasm and partly because of increased intraluminal pressure. Electron microscopy demonstrates loss of brush borders and formation of blebs on the luminal surfaces. This change often is so extensive that the proximal tubules cannot be distinguished from the distal tubules. There also is a decrease in the number of apical vacuoles and an increase in the number of large cytoplasmic vacuoles and of phagolysosomes filled with osmiophilic debris. Rough endoplasmic reticulum is more prominent, and mitochondria show a variety of nonspecific changes. "Attachment bodies" at the base of the cells, which normally consist of fine filaments, tend to aggregate into coarse bundles, and the underlying basement membrane becomes wrinkled and thickened. Important alterations are a decrease in the number of basal interdigitations, a decrease in the number of lateral processes and bizarre interdigitations with adjacent cells. As a result of these changes, cell bodies become simplified and more cuboidal. Similar alterations also occur in distal convoluted tubules and, to a lesser extent, in cortical collecting ducts.

It should be added that changes of the brush borders and of the basal and lateral interdigitations are not specific for acute tubular necrosis; such changes also occur in obstructive uropathy, tubular obstruction by casts (e.g., multiple myeloma), glomerulonephritis and acute interstitial nephritis. Regenerative changes begin within a few days and in most cases parallel the functional recovery. At first, degeneration and regeneration often coexist. Desquamated cells are replaced by flat, undifferentiated cells, which may show mitotic figures and bizarre nuclei. After some time, such cells assume a normal configuration, whereas the brush borders of the less damaged cells regenerate and the basal interdigitations are restored.

In both nephrotoxic and ischemic acute tubular necrosis, the distal tubules and cortical collecting ducts are filled with hyaline and granular casts. The latter are particularly numerous and often brownish. The casts consist primarily of precipitated Tamm-Horsfall protein mixed with varying proportions of protein derived from disintegrating tubular cells and with protein from blood plasma. Interstitial tissue is edematous and infiltrated by a moderate number of inflammatory cells, particularly at the corticomedullary junction. Peritubular capillaries often contain numerous nucleated cells. Bowman's space of the glomeruli frequently is dilated and filled with fine granular, proteinaceous material. Glomerular capillaries are partly collapsed and, on occasion, contain fibrin thrombi. Electron microscopy also demonstrates changes in the glomerular capillary walls, such as progressive loss of fine foot processes and, perhaps, a decrease in the number and alteration of shape of the endothelial fenestrae.

Recovery after acute tubular necrosis sometimes is incomplete. Tubular epithelium does not return to normal, and interstitial edema is replaced by fibrosis. In such cases, functional recovery also is incomplete and may be manifest by decreased ability to concentrate the urine and decreased functional reserve.

Incompatible Blood Transfusion

Incompatible blood transfusion is now a rare but dramatic event; it leads to hemolysis of mismatched cells, hemoglobinuria and, frequently, renal failure. Hemoglobin is only slightly toxic to tubular cells, but when hemoglobinuria is combined with shock, hypoxia, acidosis or sodium depletion, it may lead to the typical picture of acute renal failure. Other causes of hemoglobinuria include malaria (blackwater fever), paroxysmal hemoglobinuria, drug ingestion (quinine), chemical intoxication (arsine) and severe exertion; on occasion, these causes also lead to renal failure.

The color of the urine in hemoglobinuria depends on which hemoglobin derivative it contains: it is red with oxyhemoglobin, brown with methemoglobin and nearly black with reduced hemoglobin. Hemoglobinuria must be distinquished from hematuria with secondary lysis of red cells. Hemoglobin and its derivatives also color the blood plasma.

In hemoglobinuric acute renal failure, affected kidneys are enlarged and edematous and their medullae are congested and darker than the cortex. Microscopic examination reveals evidence of proximal tubular injury, as occurs in vasomotor nephropathy, as well as heavily pigmented casts in the distal tubules. The casts often are a mixture of disintegrating tubular cells and hemoglobin. The latter can be identified by proper histochemical tests.

Myoglobinuria

Myoglobin is believed to be more toxic to tubular cells than is hemoglobin, but it induces renal failure under conditions similar to those that apply to hemoglobin. Myoglobin is liberated from muscles by various types of injury; examples are trauma (crush injury), ischemia (arterial occlusion), exertion and exposure to toxins (snake venom, alcohol). However, myoglobin also is liberated in certain hereditary diseases (paroxysmal hemoglobinuria, McArdle's disease). Myoglobinuric nephropathy is similar macroscopically and microscopically to hemoglobinuric nephropathy. It may be difficult microscopically to distinguish between myoglobin and hemoglobin in tissue sections and in the plasma and urine, and immunologic methods are most useful for this purpose. In myoglobinuria, the urine also may be highly colored but, in contrast to hemoglobinuria, the serum is clear and the muscle enzyme (e.g., creatine phosphokinase) levels usually are elevated.

Acute Tubular Injury/Necrosis
Direct Tubulotoxic Injury

Fig. 10-1   Dioxane injury, experimental. Rat kidney showing vacuolation and disintegration of proximal tubular epithelial cells. (hematoxylin and eosin, ×430)

Fig. 10-2   Ethylene glycol poisoning. Tubular degeneration and oxalate crystals in tubular lumina. (hematoxylin and eosin, ×270)

Fig. 10-3   Same section as in Figure 10-2, under polarized light. (×270) (also see Chapter 11)

Fig. 10-4   Tubular vacuolation and disruption of epithelial cells in a human case, cause unknown. Patient had acute renal failure. (hematoxylin and eosin, ×270)

Fig. 10-5   Carbon tetrachloride poisoning. Partial recovery, with residual damage manifested by atrophic flat tubular epithelium and interstitial fibrosis. (hematoxylin and eosin, ×110)

Acute Vasomotor Nephropathy

Fig. 10-6   Acute vasomotor nephropathy. Renal cortex is pale; medulla is congested.

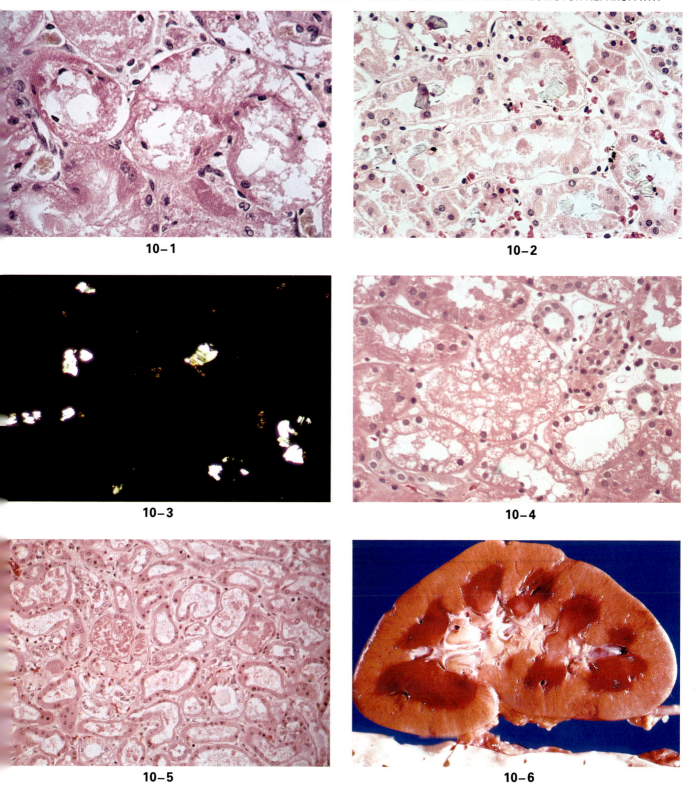

10-1

10-2

10-3

10-4

10-5

10-6

Acute Vasomotor Nephropathy

Fig. 10-7 Acute vasomotor nephropathy. Tubular dilatation, desquamation of cells and interstitial edema. (hematoxylin and eosin, × 135)

Fig. 10-8 Acute vasomotor nephropathy. Another case showing focal tubular necrosis with desquamation of cells and granular and hyaline casts in tubules. Note sparse inflammatory cells. (hematoxylin and eosin, × 270)

Fig. 10-9 Congestion and numerous nucleated cells in capillaries of renal medulla. (hematoxylin and eosin, × 270)

Fig. 10-10 Regenerating tubular epithelial cells showing mitotic activity. (hematoxylin and eosin, × 430)

Hemoglobinuric Nephropathy

Fig. 10-11 Incompatible blood transfusion. Necrotic epithelial and granular casts in tubules of renal cortex. (hematoxylin and eosin, × 110)

Fig. 10-12 Same case as in Figure 10-11. Remnants of desquamated cells and brownish granular material in collecting duct. (hematoxylin and eosin, × 270)

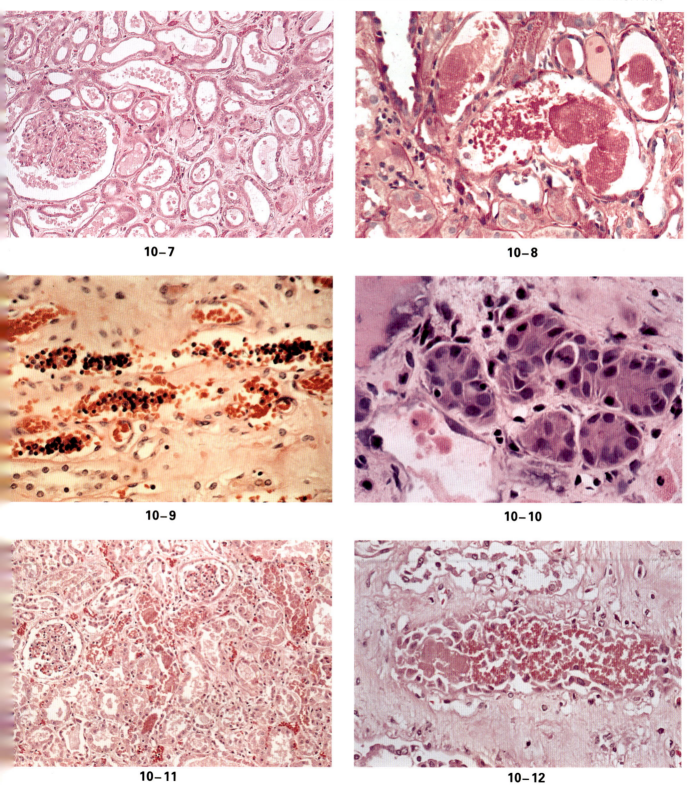

10–7

10–8

10–9

10–10

10–11

10–12

Hemoglobinuric Nephropathy

Fig. 10-13   Another section from the case shown in Figure 10-12, stained for hemoglobin, which is bluish-black. (benzidine, ×270)

Fig. 10-14   Another case of incompatible blood transfusion. Compacted hemoglobin cast filling tubular lumen. (hematoxylin and eosin, ×270)

Myoglobinuric Nephropathy

Fig. 10-15   Extensive necrosis of muscle following crush injury. (hematoxylin and eosin, ×270)

Fig. 10-16   Brownish discoloration and desquamation of tubular cells in renal medulla. (hematoxylin and eosin, ×430)

Fig. 10-17   Desquamation of tubular cells and precipitation of myoglobin in lumina. (periodic acid-Schiff, ×220)

Fig. 10-18   Same case as in Figure 10-17, stained for myoglobin. Desquamated cells and myoglobin precipitate stain dark brown. (immunoperoxidase, ×220)

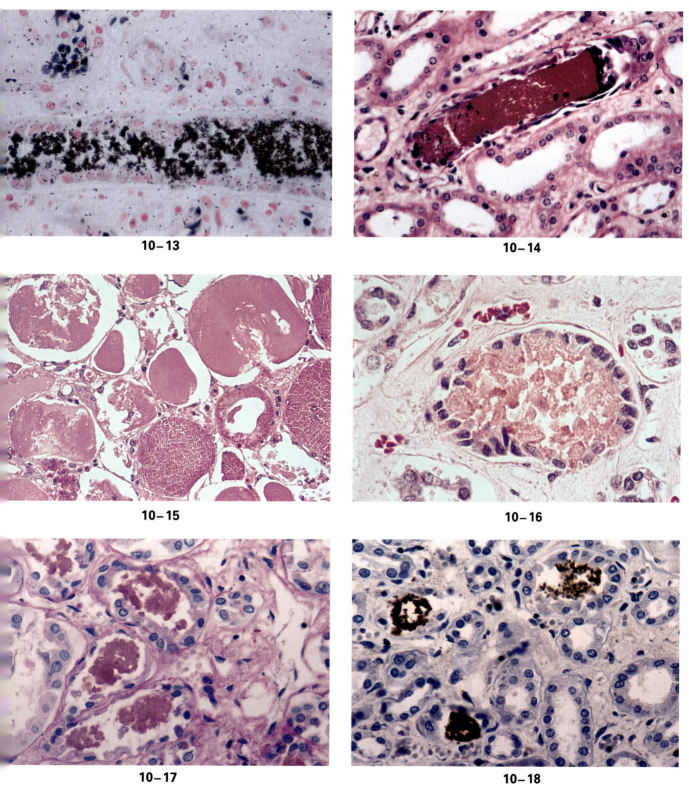

10–13

10–14

10–15

10–16

10–17

10–18

Direct Tubulotoxic Injury

Fig. 10-19 Dioxane intoxication, experimental. Same animal as in Figure 10-1. Large merging vacuoles and disruption of cytoplasm of proximal tubular cells. (electron micrograph, ×3600)

Fig. 10-20 Better-preserved tubular cell from another animal showing striking hyperplasia of smooth endoplasmic reticulum. (electron micrograph, ×16,000)

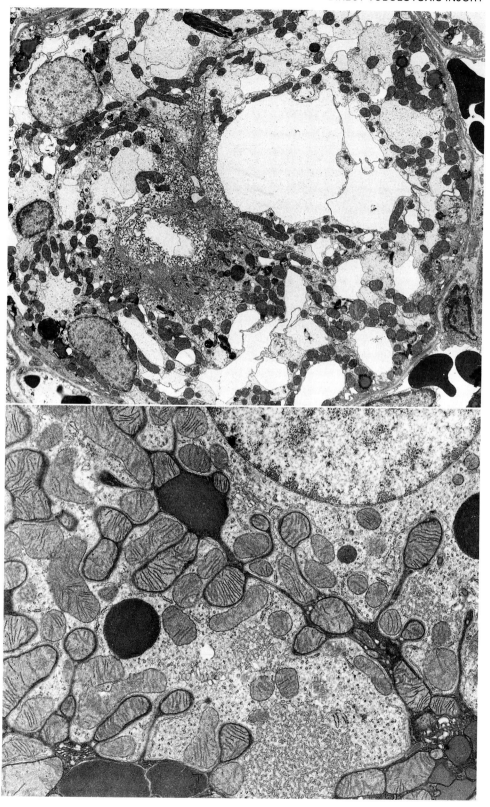

Direct Tubulotoxic Injury

Fig. 10-21 Patient with acute renal failure and toxic vacuolar nephropathy. Same case as in Figure 10-4. Large vacuoles filling cytoplasm of proximal tubular cell. (electron micrograph, ×5500)

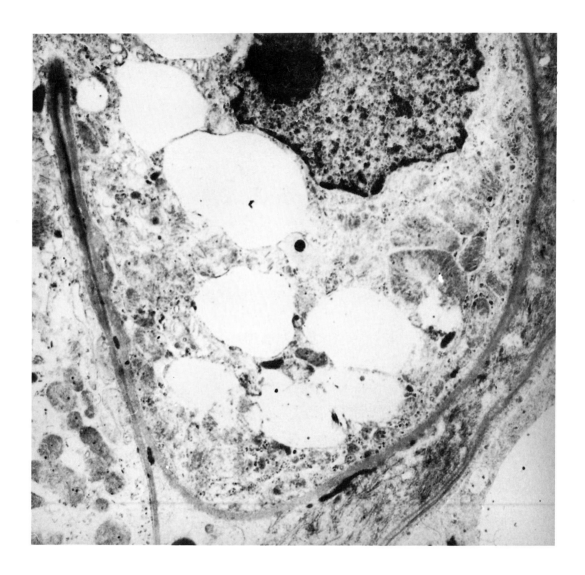

Direct Tubulotoxic Injury

Fig. 10-22 Degeneration of proximal tubular cells. Large lysosomes and numerous myeloid bodies are seen in cytoplasm. (electron micrograph, ×6000)

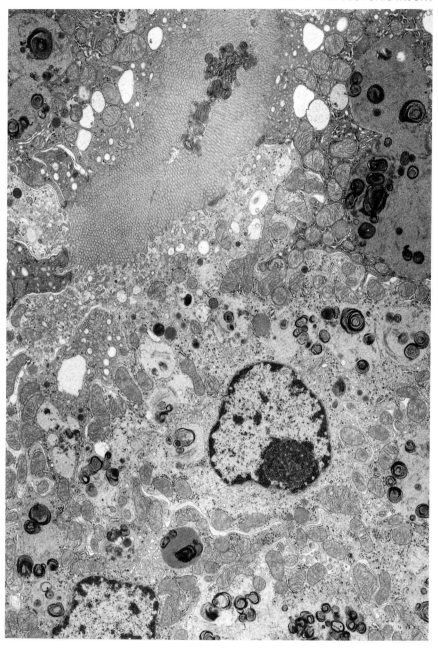

Direct Tubulotoxic Injury

Fig. 10-23 Higher magnification of the specimen shown in Figure 10-22. Complex myeloid body in the cell cytoplasm. (electron micrograph, ×28,000)

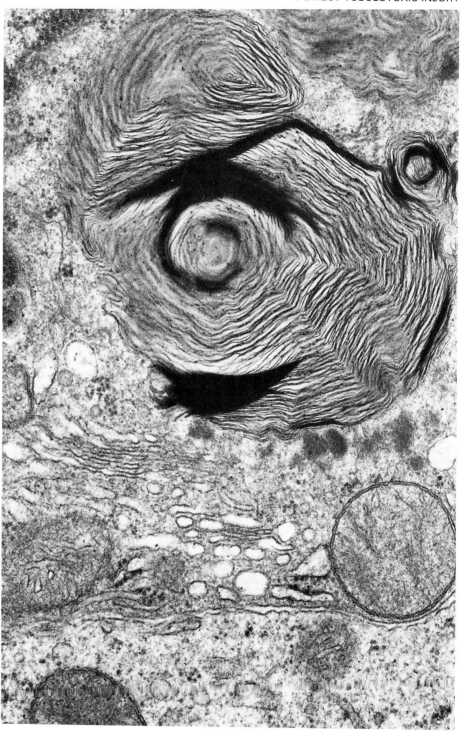

Acute Vasomotor Nephropathy

Fig. 10-24 Acute renal failure in a child. Proximal convoluted tubule with deficient brush borders, simplified cell shape and contracted basal attachment bodies of cytoskeleton (arrows), which result in the basement membrane wrinkles. (electron micrograph, ×3200)

Fig. 10-25 Same case as in Figure 10-24. Luminal surface of proximal tubule showing sparse, stubby microvilli, small blebs and long or stubby cilia. (scanning electron micrograph, ×4000)

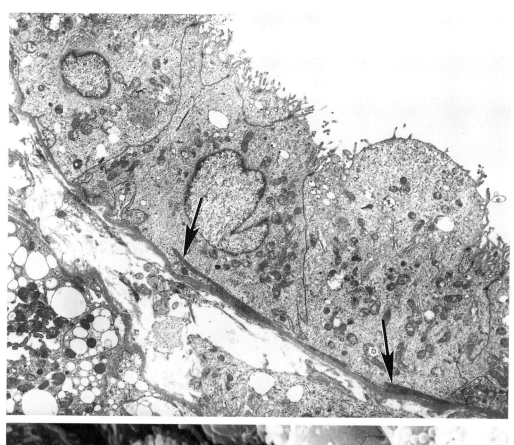

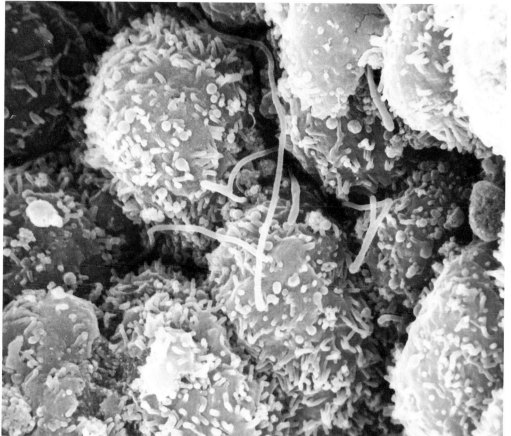

CHAPTER 11

Tubular and Tubulo-interstitial Nephropathy
Caused by Metabolic Disturbances

Tubular and Tubulo-interstitial Nephropathy Caused by Metabolic
Disturbances

Hypercalcemic Nephropathy

This type of nephropathy accompanies or is secondary to hypercalcemia and results in variable degrees of impairment of renal function (ranging from inability to concentrate the urine to progressive renal insufficiency) and, frequently, deposition of calcium salts in the kidneys (nephrocalcinosis). Stones can form within the urinary tract. There are a variety of causes of hypercalcemic nephropathy.

Clinical Manifestations: Hypercalcemic nephropathy can arise from two main types of disorder: increased absorption or ingestion of calcium (e.g., vitamin D overdosage, idiopathic hypercalcemia, milk-alkali syndrome, sarcoidosis) and skeletal depletion of calcium (hyperparathyroidism, neoplastic lytic lesions of bones, immobilization of skeleton, hyperthyroidism). In these conditions, an elevated serum level of total calcium or of ionized calcium is found, except in secondary hyperparathyroidism, in which calcium levels are slightly decreased or normal. In patients with a low serum level of protein, the level of ionized calcium may be raised even though the serum level of total calcium is normal. Hypercalciuria reflects an overload of calcium in the kidneys.

Vitamin D overdosage may be asymptomatic, or there may be a history of muscle weakness,

thirst and fatigue, sometimes accompanied by vomiting, abdominal pain and psychiatric disorders. There are two forms of idiopathic hypercalciuria. The infantile type, which affects children and infants who suffer from proteinuria and/or polyuria or dwarfism and, in severe cases, causes malformations of the face and facial bones, carries a poor prognosis. The adult type, which is manifest during adulthood, occurs more often in men than in women. This type is manifested only by an unexplained increase in the excretion of calcium. In sarcoidosis, the serum level of calcium may be elevated. In addition to renal lesions due to nephrocalcinosis and granuloma formation or accompanying glomerulonephritis, there is a direct depressing effect of the hypercalcemia on renal function, even without organic damage. Primary hyperparathyroidism caused by tumor or hyperplasia of a parathyroid gland may be asymptomatic or may be manifested by recurrent stone formation. Most patients, however, complain of thirst, weakness, polyuria and signs of progressive renal insufficiency. This condition occasionally starts during the second or third decade, and the peak incidence is in the fifth and sixth decades. Secondary hyperparathyroidism as a consequence of chronic renal failure is characterized by elevated serum levels of phosphate and alkaline phosphatase and by a normal or decreased serum level of calcium. Neoplastic lytic lesions of bones leading to hypercalcemic nephropathy are caused mostly by bone erosion but occasionally are due as well to the action of a substance similar in effect to parathyroid hormone, which is found in the tissues of patients with metastatic cancer.

Light Microscopic Findings: In hematoxylin and eosin-stained sections, basophilic deposits of calcium are observed in the cortex and medulla in an irregular distribution. There are two types deposit. Homogeneous, or band-shaped, calcifications may be seen in the basement membranes of tubules and glomerular capsules or obsolescent glomeruli. Less frequently, walls of small arteries may show amorphous deposits that stain dark blue with hematoxylin and eosin and dark brown with periodic acid-Schiff. Also, polycyclically outlined clumps of an irregular plaquelike material that consists of ring-like structures may be observed in association with tubules (proximal, distal, thin part of loops of Henle, collecting ducts). Large clumps often protrude through epithelial walls into the tubular lumina. It is therefore possible that a special cutting plane can falsely demonstrate deposits within the tubular lumina. Polycyclic clumps react strongly with von Kossa's stain, and foreign body giant cells sometimes surround clumps of calcium.

In addition to, but independent from, the irregularly distributed calcium deposits are areas of normal parenchyma alternating with interstitial fibrosis and tubular atrophy. Atrophic tubules may be surrounded by several basement membrane layers and/or have mucoid layers in between. Fibrotic areas may contain foci of lymphocytes. Glomeruli are unchanged or secondarily altered in fibrotic areas by fibrous thickening of Bowman's capsule, whereas in most cases capillary tufts are unaffected or affected only slightly, except in areas of scar formation, in which glomeruli are obsolete.

Electron Microscopic Findings: Calcium deposits are always found in tubular basement membranes or interstitial connective tissue. The following types can be found: focal deposits of an amorphous, electron-dense material in split basement membranes and (poly-)cyclic deposits with a dark (black and gray) layered outer zone and a light inner zone, which sometimes include bizarre linear figures or dark cluster-like patterns.

There also are intracellular deposits: large dense granules in matrices of mitochondria and in lysosomal vacuoles of proximal tubules.

Urate Nephropathy

Renal damage due to urate deposition is known as urate nephropathy. The following two types can be distinguished: chronic renal changes in primary and secondary gout, which are characterized by interstitial urate-containing granulomata (tophi) and/or intratubular urate deposition, combined with interstitial fibrosis and a variety of nonspecific lesions; and acute urate overload of the kidneys as a consequence of a rapid and excessive increase in the excretion of uric acid (during the first days of life and during other periods of rapid breakdown of cells, for example, in myeloproliferative disorders, cancer and, especially, during cytotoxic therapy). Both types of urate nephropathy, can be accompanied by formation of urate stones and gravel in the urinary tract.

Clinical Features: Patients who suffer from primary gout (as a genetically determined disorder of purine metabolism with hyperuricemia) may show progressive deterioration of renal function with age (after 40 years). Hypertension and atherosclerosis develop simultaneously. In spite of the raised serum level of uric acid, daily urinary excretion of urate may be normal. Advances in the management of gout have decreased the incidence of urate nephropathy as a concomitant feature, and fatalities due to gout nephropathy are now uncommon.

Secondary gout is the term used for the complications of any underlying disease that leads to hyperuricemia and a condition similar to primary gout. Such diseases include myeloproliferative disorders (e.g., leukemia, lymphoma, myeloma, polycythemia vera), chronic renal insufficiency and Lesch-Nyhan syndrome, which results from complete or partial deficiency of hypoxanthine-guanine phosphoribosyltransferase.

Acute overload of the kidneys with uric acid occurs when a sudden and excessive breakdown of nuclei-containing cells gives rise to a massive release of nucleic acids. This phenomenon occurs during the first days of life (due to breakdown of extramedullary erythropoiesis) and in patients with tumors (e.g., myeloproliferative) or other diseases, spontaneously or during therapy with cytostatic drugs. These conditions may occur without deterioration of kidney function, although temporary impairment of kidney function, may result in oliguria, and there may be urate gravel formation in the urinary tract. According to a recent study, patients with gout in whom chronic renal disease develops have been ingesting increased amounts of lead, suggesting that lead may play a part in chronic gouty nephropathy.

Macroscopic and Light and Electron Microscopic Findings: Chronic Renal Changes in Primary and Secondary Gout: Macroscopic examination usually shows that the kidneys are smaller than normal. Their surfaces display an irregular granularity and coarse scars. The cortex is reduced in width, and white spots and/or radiating lines may be seen in the medulla.

The pyramids often are scarred and deformed, and the pelvis is distorted and dilated, especially if it contains urate stones.

Microscopic studies reveal a characteristic feature, an interstitial deposit of radially oriented crystals of sodium urate that are best seen in alcohol-fixed specimens. The deposits stain deep blue with hematoxylin and eosin and exhibit birefringence with polarized light. In formol-fixed tissues, the crystals are mostly dissolved, and only empty lacunae remain. There may be an amorphous, faint blue material that contains a few delicate crystals. These deposits are surrounded by mononuclear inflammatory cells and giant cells with accompanying tubular sclerosis and atrophy.

There also are rectangular or irregularly shaped, doubly refractile crystals in the tubular lumina. Crystal deposits are found mainly in the medulla and are located in intact or degenerating collecting tubules.

Gout granulomas are rarely seen in the renal cortex, an important point to remember in making a diagnosis on the basis of biopsy material.

In most cases, there are few urate granulomas in the kidneys, and this finding does not satisfactorily explain the spectrum of alterations that typically are observed; focal or more or less diffuse interstitial fibrosis (with or without focal lymphocytic infiltrates) and tubular atrophy, partly with dilated lumina that contain condensed protein, is the common finding. Glomeruli show widening of the mesangium and, sometimes, thickening of capillaries, with an increase in the mesangial matrix and accumulation of a matrix-like substance in the lamina rara interna, as seen with the electron microscope. Blood vessels may show arteriolosclerosis. Doubtless, the chronic renal damage seen in gout is the result of the interaction of many changes, including urate-induced fibrosis, obstruction of nephrons in deeper areas of the kidney and reactions of the cortical parenchyma combined with inflammatory changes as well as vascular alteration.

Changes in Acute Urate Overload: Macroscopic examination reveals a characteristic feature, a golden-yellow radial striation in the medulla or pyramids (so-called uric acid infarct). In such cases, microscopic studies demonstrate rounded crystals of ammonium urate in the lumina of distal tubules and collecting ducts, whose epithelial walls may be intact or focally disrupted.

Oxalate Nephropathy

This condition occurs when there is deposition of calcium oxalate crystals, resulting in renal fibrosis and atrophy. It is caused by a congenital enzyme deficiency or by endogenous or exogenous poisoning.

Clinical and Pathogenetic Features: *Primary hyperoxaluria:* Two types have been identified; both are the result of enzyme deficiencies. Type I is caused by an absence of 2-hydroxy-3-oxoadipate carboxylase, which leads to increases in glyoxylate and glycolate levels. This type is inherited as an autosomal recessive character. In type II, there is a deficiency of the enzyme glyoxylate transferase, whose inheritance is not yet clear. Both metabolic disorders lead to excessive synthesis of oxalate and glycolate, independent of the intake of oxalate with food. Large amounts of oxalate are excreted in the urine.

In infants, the disease presents with microhematuria and/or slight proteinuria. Detection of oxalate and glycolate in excessive quantities in the urine establishes the diagnosis. Terminal renal insufficiency often develops insidiously.

Secondary hyperoxaluria can develop as a consequence of poisoning with ethylene glycol (antifreeze), anesthesia with methoxyflurane or deficiency of pyridoxine (vitamine B_6).

In uremia, especially when there is severe acidosis, numerous oxalate crystals are found within the renal tubules. Oxalosis may occur in renal transplants.

Macroscopic Findings: In the end stage of primary hyperoxaluria, the kidneys may be smaller than normal, and the surface appears irregularly granular and scarred. The cortex is reduced in width and may show crystalline aggregates discernible with a hand lens. The distended pelvis often contains several stones.

Light and Electron Microscopic Findings: Histologic sections of contracted kidneys show severe interstitial fibrosis with tubular atrophy and varying degrees of glomerular obsolescence. Arteries are thickened and often obliterated. Tubular epithelium often is absent. Instead of intact tubules, one finds many irregularly defined holes in paraffin-embedded sections, which are the result of loss of crystals during sectioning. In these holes and in all types of tubules, there are abundant crystals, which may be overlooked because of their transparency in hematoxylin and eosin-stained sections.

Crystals are mostly rhomboid and often show a cluster or rosette-like arrangement. They often are combined with calcium deposits, which in hematoxylin and eosin-stained sections appear blue and which in von Kossa-stained sections stain black.

Under polarized light, the crystals are doubly refractile and show all colors of the rainbow, but predominantly yellow. With transmission electron microscopy, light crystals appear predominantly as long needles with blunt edges lying singly or in clusters or rosette-like arrangements. Usually, the epithelium and tubular basement membranes are seen in various stages of destruction. Edges of the crystals reach the interstitial space, partly surrounded by interstitial cells.

In early stages of primary hyperoxaluria, for example, in grafts that were transplanted to patients suffering from oxalosis, and in secondary hyperoxaluria, oxalate crystrals are found in widened but intact tubules. Here, most crystals are rounded and partly show globular or lamellar calcium inclusion bodies. Therefore, care should be taken to distinguish primary oxalate nephropathy from increased deposition of oxalate crystals in such cases.

Cystinosis

The reader is referred to the volume on Developmental and Hereditary Diseases.

Hypokalemic Nephropathy

The renal tubular vacuolation that develops after severe and prolonged hypokalemia is known as hypokalemic nephropathy.

Clinical Features: Hypokalemia may occur in several conditions, especially in illnesses that are accompanied by prolonged loss of fluid and electrolytes (e.g., gastrointestinal disorders with diarrhea); Bartter's syndrome; idiopathic hypokalemia (mainly in infancy, familiar and/or inherited) or symptomatic hypokalemia (after prolonged use/

abuse of laxatives or diuretics, vomiting) Conn's syndrome; secondary hyperaldosteronism or certain kidney diseases. The role of hypokalemia in inducing renal insufficiency has not been established. Clinical features are vomiting and diarrhea.

Light and Electron Microscopic Findings: The characteristic (but nonspecific) lesion consists of a more or less intense vacuolation of the proximal tubules and, in severe cases, of the distal tubules as well. Clear vacuoles may be few and distinct or so numerous and tightly packed that the cytoplasm of the epithelial cells has a foamy appearance. On electron microscopy these vacuoles are found to be of lysosomal origin, demonstrating a typical vacuolar membrane and electron-lucent contents with or without various osmiophilic inclusion bodies. In human kidney, tubules of the medullary zone remain unaffected.

Similar vacuolar phenomena also can be observed in other conditions (e.g., storage of filtered carbohydrates, such as dextran and mannitol, or in ischemia and nephrotoxic insults). The lesions are differentiated by careful clinical investigation.

Other metabolic disturbances are briefly described in the legends accompanying Figures 11-25 to 11-36.

The reader is referred to Chapter 9 for a discussion on copper deposition.

Tubular and Tubulo-interstitial Lesions
Caused by Metabolic Disturbances
Hypercalcemic Nephropathy

Fig. 11-1   Parathyroid adenoma. Large encapsulated, parathormone-secreting tumor with a high blood level of calcium.

Fig. 11-2   Bone biopsy. Same case as in Figure 11-1 showing osteitis fibrosa with bone resorption. (hematoxylin and eosin, $\times$110)

Fig. 11-3   Nephrocalcinosis due to chronic overdose of vitamin D. Cut section of kidney showing fine whitish streaks and spots in cortex as well as two small calculi in pelvis. Width of cortex is reduced in places.

Fig. 11-4   Nephrocalcinosis. Same case as in Figure 11-1. Early basophilic calcification of tubular cells and basement membranes (right upper corner). (hematoxylin and eosin, $\times$460)

Fig. 11-5   Same case as in Figure 11-4. (von Kossa's stain, $\times$270)

Fig. 11-6   Nephrocalcinosis, advanced stage. Calcification of tubules, interstitium, blood vessels and glomeruli, considerable tubular atrophy and interstitial fibrosis with inflammation. (hematoxylin and eosin, $\times$175)

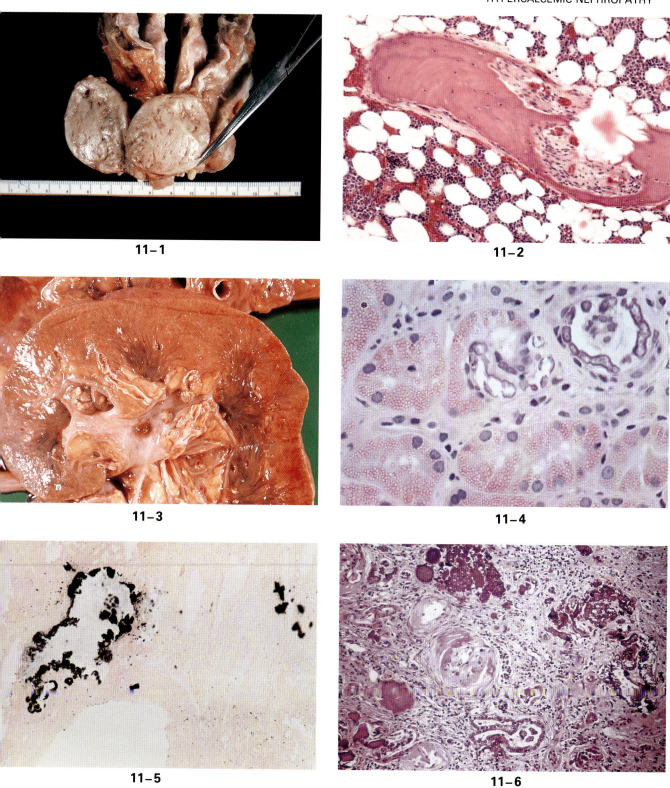

11–1

11–2

11–3

11–4

11–5

11–6

Hypercalcemic Nephropathy

Fig. 11-7   Nephrocalcinosis. Lamellar calcification of tubular basement membranes, tubular atrophy and marked interstitial fibrosis. (hematoxylin and eosin, ×430)

Fig. 11-8   Nephrocalcinosis. Foreign body giant-cell reaction to calcium deposits in tubular epithelium in a case of metastatic carcinoma of bones. (hematoxylin and eosin, ×700)

Urate Nephropathy

Fig. 11-9   Urate nephropathy, acute. Precipitation of urates in the newborn (so-called uric acid infarcts). Cut section of kidney showing golden-yellow radial streaks in medulla and papillae.

Fig. 11-10   Same case as in Figure 11-9. Rounded, birefringent crystals of ammonium urate in lumen of medullary duct. (absolute alcohol fixation, hematoxylin and eosin, polarization microscopy, ×700)

Fig. 11-11   Urate nephropathy. Urate crystals surrounded by granulomatous inflammation. (absolute alcohol fixation, hematoxylin and eosin, ×270)

Fig. 11-12   Same section as in Figure 11-11. Birefringent urate crystals. (absolute alcohol fixation, polarization microscopy, ×270)

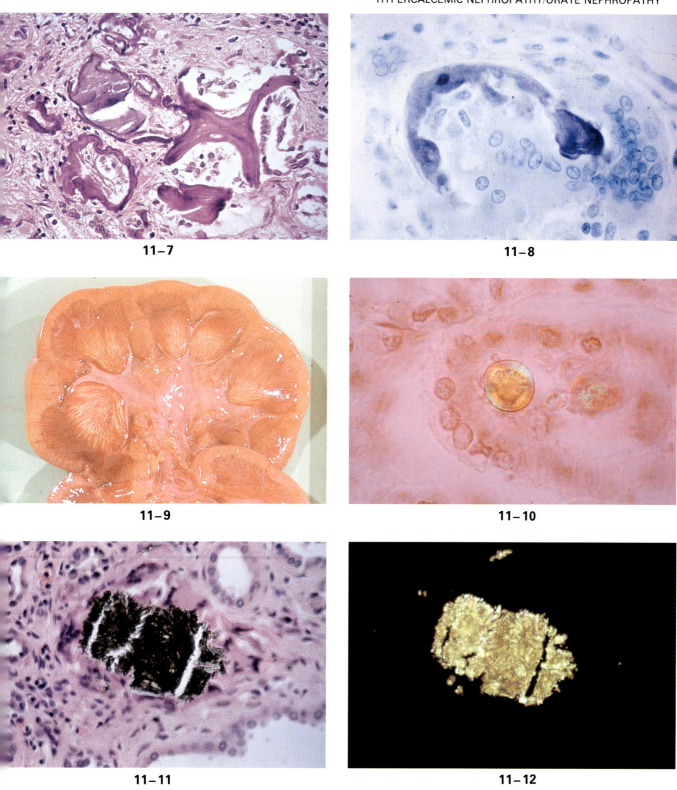

11–7

11–8

11–9

11–10

11–11

11–12

Urate Nephropathy/Oxalate Nephropathy

Fig. 11-13 Urate nephropathy, chronic. Granulomas surrounding spaces formerly filled by urate crystals. Severe tubular atrophy, chronic interstitial inflammation and fibrosis also are seen. (aqueous formaldehyde fixation, hematoxylin and eosin, ×110)

Oxalate Nephropathy

Fig. 11-14 Oxalate nephropathy, primary oxalosis. Contracted granular kidney with scattered small cortical cysts and whitish spots and small streaks in cortex and medulla.

Fig. 11-15 Oxalate nephropathy, primary oxalosis. Numerous transparent crystals in tubular lumina and focal destruction of tubular epithelium. (hematoxylin and eosin, ×350)

Fig. 11-16 Same case as in Figure 11-15. Bundles of birefringent oxalate crystals in tubular lumina. (polarization microscopy, ×350)

Fig. 11-17 Oxalate nephropathy, primary oxalosis, advanced stage. Severe tubular atrophy, interstitial fibrosis, chronic inflammation and glomerular sclerosis. (periodic acid-Schiff, ×170)

Fig. 11-18 Oxalate nephropathy, primary oxalosis. Massive deposition of oxalate crystals and destruction of renal parenchyma. (hematoxylin and eosin, ×110)

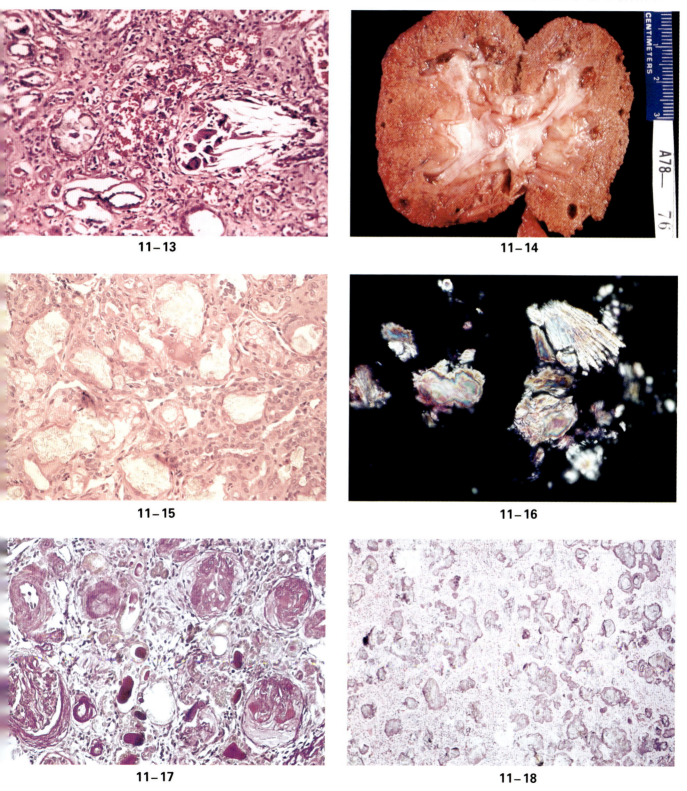

11–13

11–14

11–15

11–16

11–17

11–18

Oxalate Nephropathy

Fig. 11-19 Same section as in Figure 11-18, under polarized light. (×110)

Fig. 11-20 Oxalate nephropathy, secondary renal oxalosis in a renal transplant, probably following methoxyflurane anesthesia. Oxalate crystals in tubular lumina and epithelial cells. (hematoxylin and eosin, polarization microscopy, ×135)

Fig. 11-21 Oxalate nephropathy, secondary renal oxalosis after therapeutic infusion of xylitol (pentose alcohol). Radially arranged oxalate crystals in proximal tubule. (hematoxylin and eosin, ×700)

Fig. 11-22 Oxalate nephropathy, secondary renal oxalosis in a case of chronic renal failure. Crystals of calcium oxalate ("leucine-like" crystals) in tubular lumen. (hematoxylin and eosin, ×280)

Hypokalemic Nephropathy

Fig. 11-23 Hypokalemic nephropathy, early stage. Fine vacuoles in proximal tubular epithelial cells. (hematoxylin and eosin, ×480)

Fig. 11-24 Hypokalemic nephropathy, advanced stage. Large intracytoplasmic vacuoles displacing nuclei of tubular epithelial cells. (hematoxylin and eosin, ×430)

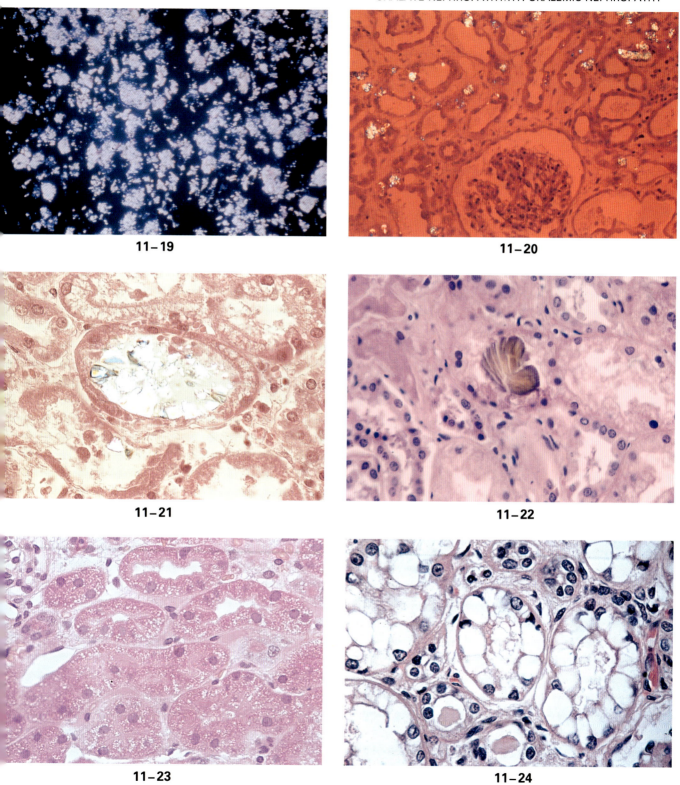

11–19

11–20

11–21

11–22

11–23

11–24

Vacuolar Change (osmotic nephropathy)

Fig. 11-25   Vacuolar change (osmotic nephropathy) after intravenous administration of mannitol. Fine vacuoles filling cytoplasm of proximal tubular cells. (hematoxylin and eosin, ×460)

Glycogen Deposition

Fig. 11-26   Glycogen deposition. Vacuolation of proximal tubular cells. Cell cytoplasm appears "washed out." (hematoxylin and eosin, ×460)

Fig. 11-27   Same case as in Figure 11-26. Periodic acid-Schiff stain shows abundant glycogen deposits. (×460)

Fatty Change

Fig. 11-28   Fatty change. Fine vacuolation of proximal tubular cells in a newborn. (hematoxylin and eosin, ×540)

Fig. 11-29   Fatty change. Numerous fat droplets in tubular cells. (frozen section, oil red O, ×430)

Hyaline Droplet Degeneration

Fig. 11-30   Large hyaline droplets in proximal tubular cells. Adjacent tubules show considerable degeneration. Patient with disseminated intravascular coagulation and acute renal failure. (periodic acid-Schiff, ×430)

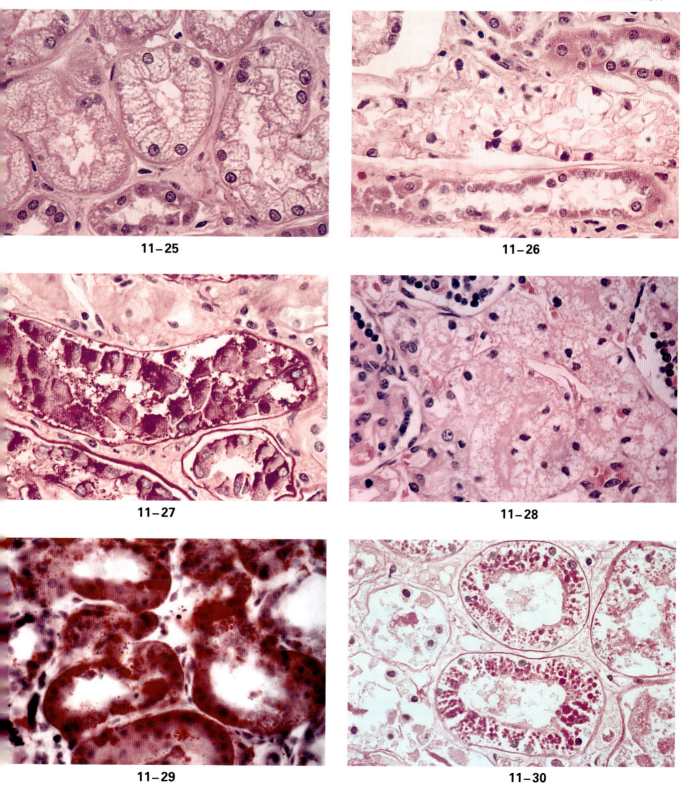

11-25

11-26

11-27

11-28

11-29

11-30

Bile Nephrosis

Fig. 11-31 Bile nephrosis. Bile staining of kidney involving cortex, medulla and papillae.

Fig. 11-32 Bile nephrosis. Bile-stained casts, bile staining and degeneration of tubular cells. (hematoxylin and eosin, ×270)

Fig. 11-33 Bile nephrosis. Greenish bile casts in tubular lumina. (hematoxylin and eosin, ×400)

Iron Deposition

Fig. 11-34 "Blue kidney." Massive deposits of hemosiderin in a patient with aortic valve prosthesis and secondary hemolytic anemia. (Prussian blue, ×80)

Melanuria

Fig. 11-35 Widely metastasizing malignant melanoma with melanuria. Melanin deposits in renal glomerulus. (hematoxylin and eosin, ×270)

Fig. 11-36 Same case as in Figure 11-35. Melanin deposits in tubular cells. (eosin, ×220)

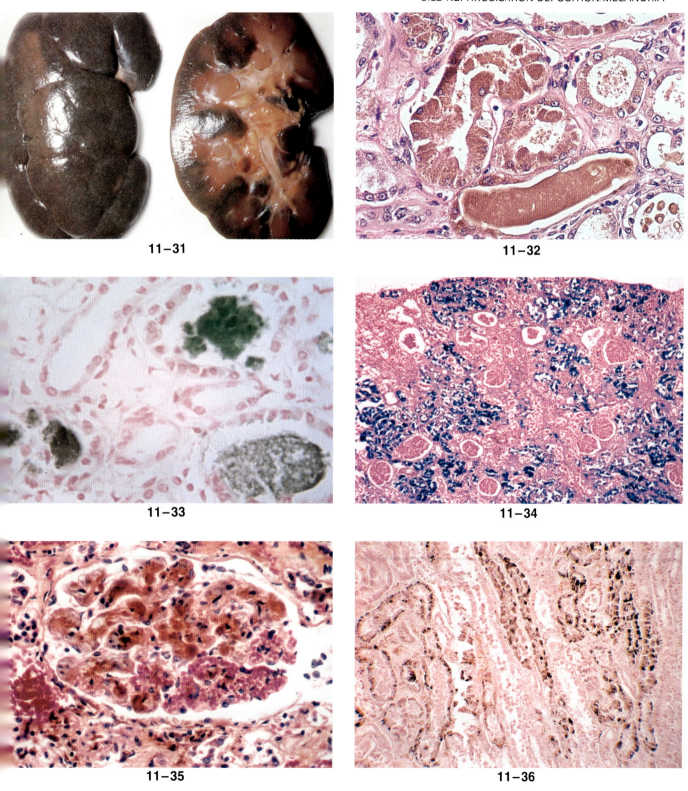

11-31

11-32

11-33

11-34

11-35

11-36

Nephrocalcinosis

Fig. 11-37 Nephrocalcinosis in experimental hypercalcemia. Early mitochondrial calcification in the shape of dark granules and rings. (electron micrograph, ×26,000)

Fig. 11-38 Nephrocalcinosis in experimental hypercalcemia. Early scalloped calcium deposits in tubular basement membranes. (electron micrograph, ×48,000)

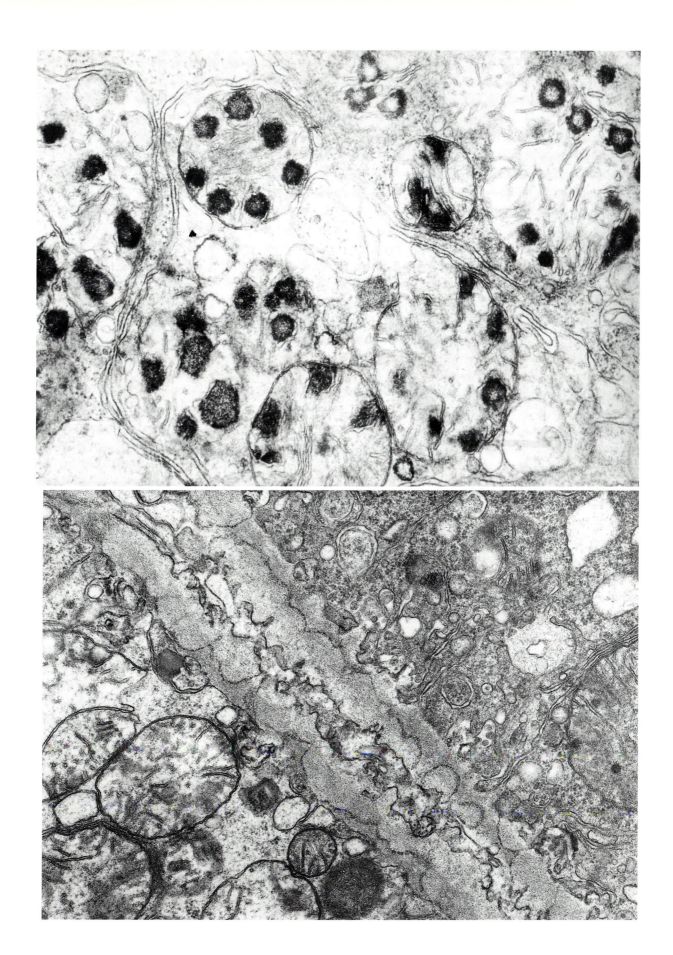

Nephrocalcinosis

Fig. 11-39 Nephrocalcinosis, human. Dense granules in lysosomal vacuoles of tubular epithelial cell. (electron micrograph, ×36,000)

Fig. 11-40 Nephrocalcinosis. Polycyclic calcified structure in renal interstitium. Interconnected rounded structures with light inner zone containing irregular fragments, outlined by narrow peripheral zone of alternating darker and lighter layers. (electron micrograph, ×11,000)

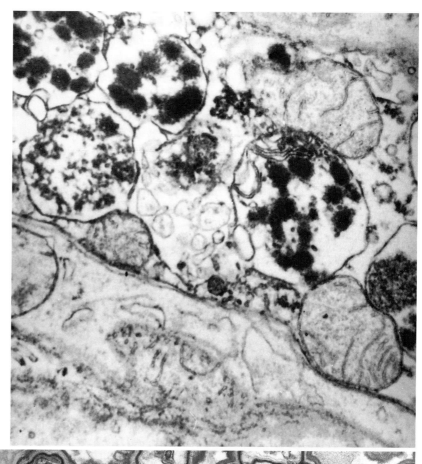

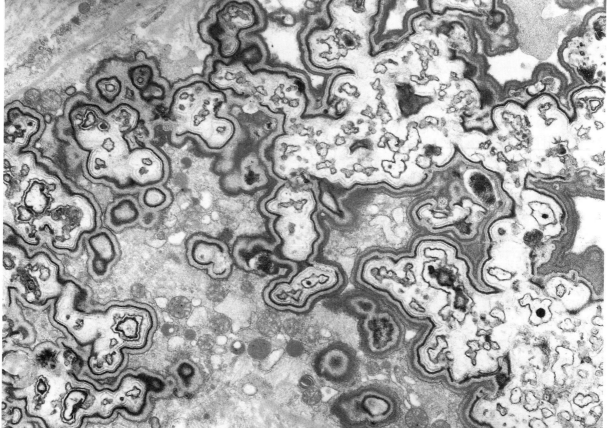

Nephrocalcinosis

Fig. 11-41 Nephrocalcinosis, human. Polycyclic calcified body with layered outer zone and dark center showing fine radial "spokes." (electron micrograph, ×44,000)

Oxalate Nephropathy

Fig. 11-42 Oxalate nephropathy, primary oxalosis. Deposition of oxalate crystals in tubules with destruction of epithelial lining. (electron micrograph, ×10,000)

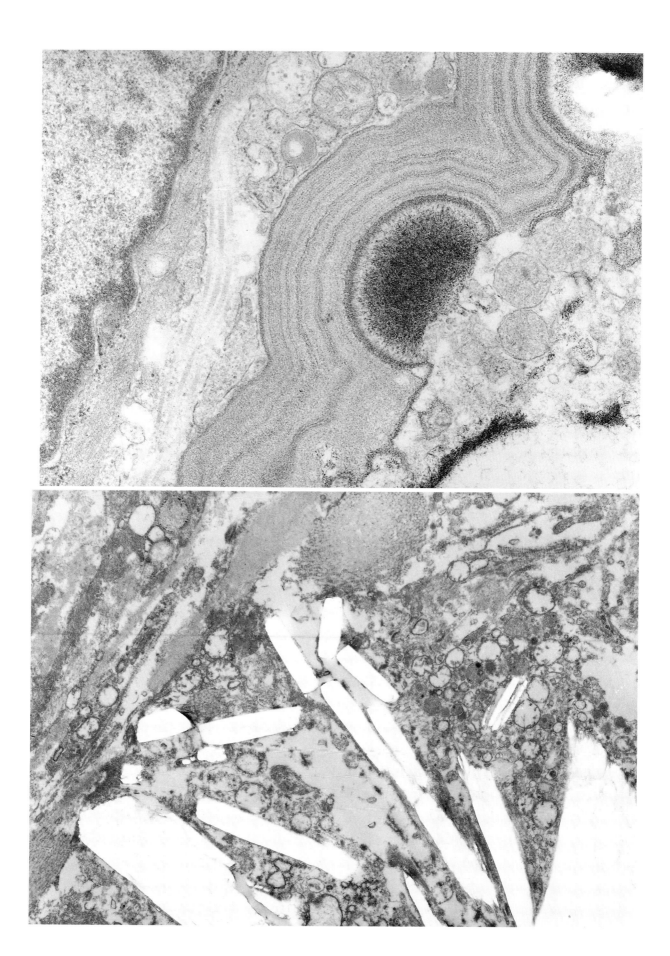

Oxalate Nephropathy

Fig. 11-43   Oxalate nephropathy, primary oxalosis. Higher magnification of a better preserved crystal showing fine tubular structures. (electron micrograph, ×76,100)

Fig. 11-44   Oxalate nephropathy, secondary renal oxalosis. Same case as in Figure 11-20. "Soft x-ray" picture of removed renal transplant.

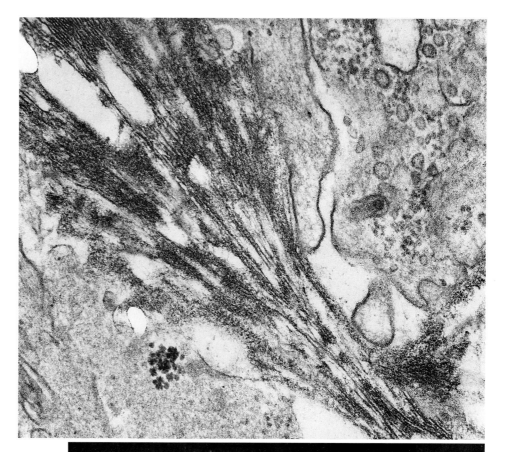

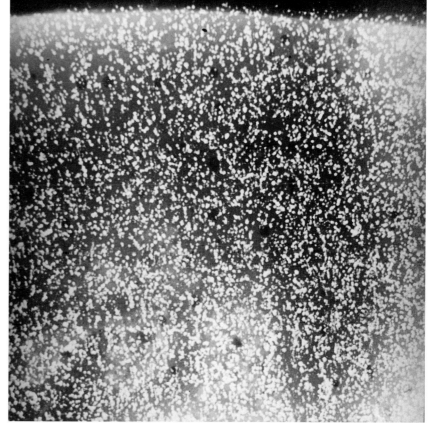

Hypokalemic Nephropathy/Fatty Tubular Degeneration

Fig. 11-45   Hypokalemic nephropathy, early stage. Proximal tubular epithelial cells. Lysosomal vacuoles containing electron-lucent material and small osmiophilic inclusions. (electron micrograph, ×28,000)

Fig. 11-46   Fatty degeneration. Needle-like crystals of fatty acids and lipid globules in cytoplasm of proximal tubular cell. (electron micrograph, ×2000)

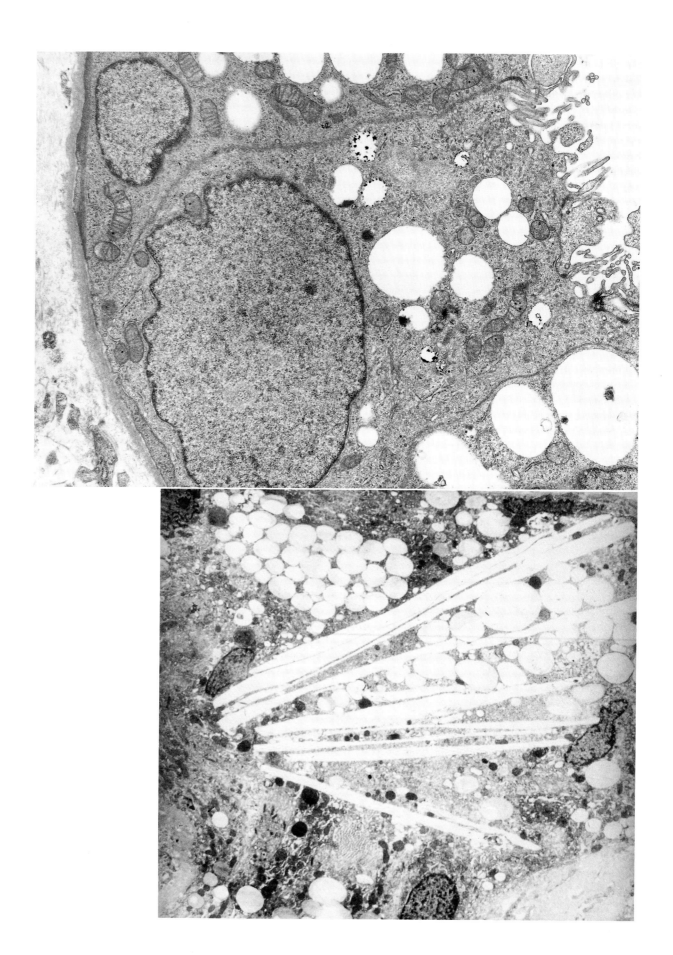

CHAPTER 12

Hereditary Renal Tubulo-interstitial Disorders
Tubulo-interstitial Nephritis Associated with
Neoplastic Disorders

Hereditary Renal Tubulo-interstitial Disorders
Tubulo-interstitial Nephritis Associated with Neoplastic Disorders

Hereditary Renal Tubulo-interstitial Disorders

Medullary cystic disease (juvenile nephronophthisis) (see volume on Developmental and Hereditary Renal Diseases)
Familial interstitial nephritis of unkonwn etiologic basis (see volume on Developmental and Hereditary Renal Diseases)
Alport's syndrome (see volume on Glomerular Diseases)

Tubulo-interstitial Nephritis Associated with Neoplastic Disorders

Plasma Cell Dyscrasias

This term covers a spectrum of diseases, which includes solitary myeloma of bone, soft tissue plasmacytoma, multiple myeloma, plasma cell leukemia and Waldenström's macroglobulinemia. There is uncontrolled proliferation of monoclonal plasma cells or related cell types with extensive disease. High levels of one immunoglobulin (M protein) and/or one of its constituent polypeptide chains are found in the blood and/or urine. Additional light or heavy chains also are synthesized, along with the complete immunoglobulins, but in some cases only light chains are found (light-chain disease). The light (L) chains are either kappa (κ) or lambda (λ), and the free light chains (Bence Jones proteins) are small and easily excreted in the urine.

Myeloma Kidney

The renal changes that occur in multiple myeloma, especially precipitation of lamellated proteins as casts in tubules, and associated tubular epithelial changes constitute myeloma kidney.

Clinical and Pathogenetic Features: Approximately 50% to 90% of Bence Jones (light chain) proteins are broken down rapidly by an endogenous catabolic process, mainly in the kidneys. The remaining Bence Jones proteins, which are small molecules (molecular weight, 22,000 or 44,000), are filtered and then absorbed and catabolized by tubular cells. Thus, patients who have multiple myeloma in association with renal disease have a significantly reduced rate of catabolism of Bence Jones proteins.

Bence Jones proteinuria is associated with an increased incidence (more than 50%) of renal insufficiency in patients with myeloma. Precipitation of Bence Jones proteins within renal tubules leads to renal obstruction and tubular damage. The latter may be due to mechanical pressure or the toxic effect of light chains on the cells. Intratubular casts are formed by combination of Bence Jones proteins with urinary Tamm-Horsfall protein at acidic pH. The casts tend to obstruct the tubular lumina and induce an inflammatory reaction. Clinically, renal failure develops insidiously and usually progresses slowly over several months or years. In some patients, it manifests as acute renal failure with oliguria, often precipitated by dehydration, administration of nephrotoxic antibiotics or intravenous infusion of x-ray contrast media.

Macroscopic Findings: The kidneys vary in appearance. They may be normal in size and color but more often are enlarged and pale, although they occasionally are shrunken due to scarring and atrophy of the renal cortex.

Light Microscopic Findings: Large casts are found principally in distal convoluted and collecting tubules. The casts may be homogeneous and eosinophilic or polychromatic or lamellated and often are surrounded by multinucleated giant cells formed by epithelial cells or by macrophages. Granulomas may extend into adjoining interstitium.

The cytoplasm of proximal tubular cells may contain large hyaline protein droplets or needle-like inclusion bodies that stain pink with hematoxylin and eosin and purple with phosphotungstic acid hematoxylin. Tubules are commonly dilated, and epithelium surrounding the casts is atrophic and sometimes necrotic, so that the casts are in direct contact with thickened basement mem-

branes or even penetrate into surrounding interstitium. Tubular basement membranes may contain rounded, laminated and basophilic calcium salt deposits. There is interstitial fibrosis and lymphocytic infiltration in areas of tubular atrophy. Arteries may show intimal thickening and hyaline arteriolosclerosis. Focal collections of immature plasma cells, amyloid deposits and obstructive focal pyelonephritis may be found.

Electron Microscopic Findings: Glomeruli may show focal basement membrane thickening and focal subendothelial deposits of coarse granular material (see volume on Glomerular Diseases).

Tubular casts have a varied composition: finely granular material of moderate electron density, coarse granular material of high electron density and, often, fine fibrils. Fibrils measure approximately 10 μm in diameter and tend to form parellel bundles. Casts also may contain bundles of electron-dense crystals, varying from rectangles to fine needles.

Tubular cells have distended endoplasmic reticulum and swollen mitochondria. Cast material, including fibrils and crystals, may be found in the cytoplasm lying free or within membrane-bound vesicles. Tubular basement membranes are thickened and focally split. They may contain cell organelles, granular bodies (20 to 100 μm in diameter) and occasional myelin figures. Many collagen fibrils are present in interstitial tissue.

Immunofluorescence Microscopic Findings: The casts contain immunoglobulins, complement, albumin and, in many instances, fibrinogen. Tamm-Horsfall protein is almost invariably present. Usually, both light chains, κ and λ, are found, even in cases in which only one is excreted in the urine, but sometimes the predominant staining is only for the type of light chain associated with the 7S serum M components or the light chain produced by the myeloma. No autofluorescence of casts is detected in unstained sections.

Light-Chain Nephropathy

Although most manifestations of myeloma kidney are produced by light-chain proteins, there is a special form of disease, usually caused by κ light chains, which often manifests as Fanconi's syndrome, but also as proteinuria and renal failure. Fanconi's syndrome is characterized by renal glycosuria, aminoaciduria, phosphaturia and acidosis and is due to tubular cell damage. In children, this syndrome is hereditary (see volume on Developmental and Hereditary Renal Diseases); in adults, it is acquired and most often associated with malignant lesions, usually multiple myeloma but occasionally carcinoma of the ovary, pancreas or liver. In some patients, it appears to be idiopathic.

Clinical and Pathogenetic Features: The κ chain is reabsorbed by proximal tubular cells, in which it forms crystal-like structures within phagolysosomes. The material is apparently toxic to the tubules, interfering with their function, such as absorption of albumin, low-molecular-weight serum proteins and glucose, phosphates and bicarbonate. It may also lead to tubular degeneration and renal failure.

Microscopic Findings: Inclusion bodies are found in proximal tubular cells. Basement membranes sometimes are thickened and strongly positive with periodic acid-Schiff. On electron microscopy, tubular degeneration is found to be manifest by focal destruction of microvilli, subapical swelling and vacuolation and mitochondrial damage. The cytoplasm contains numerous rodlike, finely crystalline structures. Electron-dense deposits may be found in linear arrangement along the tubular and glomerular basement membranes. Fluorescence microscopy demontrates that such deposits consist of light chains, most often κ chains. Light chains also are demonstrable in the cell cytoplasm.

Mixed IgG-IgM Cryoglobulinemia (see Chapter 6)

This state usually gives rise to glomerular lesions, but tubules and interstitium may be involved. The tubules show atrophy, and their lumina contain casts. Variable numbers of mononuclear cells and lymphocytes may be present in the interstitium.

Waldenström's Macroglobulinemia (see volume on Glomerular Diseases)

In this lymphoproliferative neoplastic disease, there is infiltration by immature lymphoid cells of the B type, predominantly in lymphoid tissues but also in other organs. The kidneys may be involved directly by infiltrates or indirectly by secondary amyloidosis. The clinical sign of renal involvement is proteinuria, which occasionally is severe. Nephrotic syndrome may develop and terminate in renal failure. The serum level of IgM is elevated, and single light chains or cryoglobulins may be present. The urine may contain Bence Jones proteins.

Important changes are seen in glomeruli. Capillaries are distended by protein masses, which with fluorescence microscopy are found to contain IgM but which may also stain with fibrin. They are attached to capillary walls, but there are no true intramembranous deposits. Similar "thrombi" also may be seen in arterioles. Protein casts may appear in proximal and distal tubules but often are inconspicuous. Cellular atrophy is present in connection with massive casts. Interstitial infiltration by neoplastic cells is a common finding, both in the cortex and in the medulla. When amyloid deposits are present, they are mostly localized to the glomeruli. Renal changes are characteristic of the disease, although similar glomerular and tubular interstitial changes have been described in a few cases of multiple myeloma.

Leukemic and Lymphomatous Infiltration

The kidney is a common organ for leukemic infiltration, and this finding should not be mistakenly diagnosed as tubulo-interstitial nephritis. Leukemic infiltrates are found as perivascular aggregates that progressively involve the interstitium in a diffuse distribution. If cellular infiltration is heavy, it may compress and destroy the tubules.

When the infiltrates are large, they are visible macroscopically as pale gray areas, which are not well defined. With bone marrow suppression of platelets by the cancer, hemorrhage may occur in the mucosa of the renal pelves and calices.

Tubulo-interstitial Nephritis Associated with Neoplasia
Plasma Cell Dyscrasias
Myeloma Kidney

Fig. 12-1 Myeloma kidney. Dense fragmented and layered tubular casts surrounded by proliferating cells. Considerable interstitial fibrosis. (hematoxylin and eosin, ×270)

Fig. 12-2 Myeloma kidney. Tubular cast with attached multinucleated giant cell. (hematoxylin and eosin, ×430)

Fig. 12-3 Tubular casts stained with anti-lambda antiserum. (fluorescence microscopy, ×430)

Light-Chain Nephropathy

Fig. 12-4 Light-chain nephropathy. Thickening of tubular basement membranes and mild interstitial fibrosis. (periodic acid-Schiff, ×270)

Leukemic and Lymphomatous Infiltration

Fig. 12-5 Acute myeloid leukemia. Infiltration of renal interstitium by leukemic cells. (Care should be taken not to mistake such cells for inflammatory cells.) (hematoxylin and eosin, ×270)

188

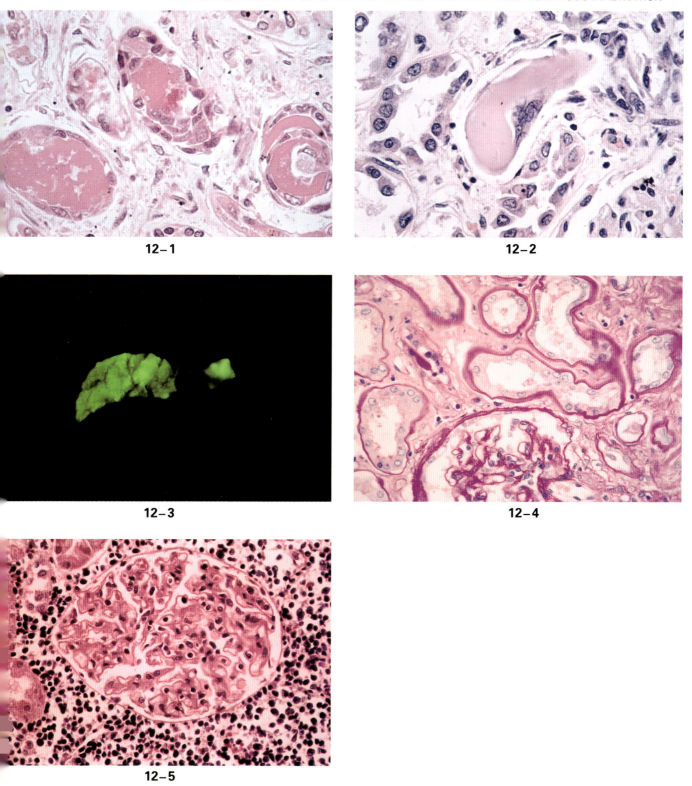

12–1

12–2

12–3

12–4

12–5

Light-Chain Nephropathy

Fig. 12-6   Light-chain nephropathy. Electron-dense linear deposits along tubular basement membranes. (electron micrograph, ×10,000)

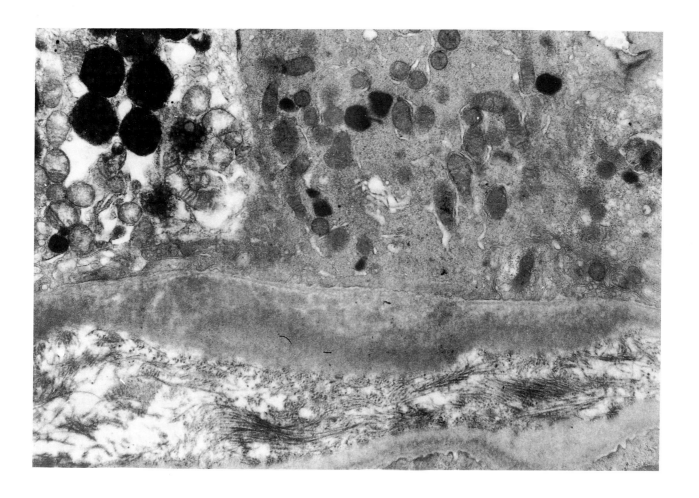

CHAPTER 13

Tubulo-interstitial Lesions in Glomerular and Vascular Diseases
End-stage Kidney

Tubulo-interstitial Lesions in Glomerular and Vascular Diseases
End-stage Kidney

Tubulo-interstitial Lesions in Glomerular and Vascular Diseases
Acute and Chronic Glomerular Diseases

Acute or active diseases of glomeruli, such as proliferative glomerulonephritis, often are accompanied by damage to tubular cells, varying from changes visible only by electron microscopy (similar to those seen in vasomotor nephropathy, see Chapter 10), to frank degeneration. Interstitial changes also are common and include edema and inflammation. The latter is especially prominent in some immunologically induced processes, such as Goodpasture's syndrome and systemic lupus erythematosus, in which immune deposits are found along tubular basement membranes and in connective tissue (see tubulo-interstitial nephritis associated with immune disorders, Chapter 6). Occasionally, inflammation is frankly necrotizing and granulomatous, as in Wegener's granulomatosis.

In diseases accompanied by massive proteinuria, hyaline (protein) droplets accumulate in tubular cells and hyaline casts form in their lumina. On occasion, the casts are large and very numerous, leading to intratubular obstruction and renal insufficiency. Lipiduria is a frequent concomitant of massive proteinuria (e.g., in nephrotic syndrome) but may occur as an independent phenomenon in cases of severe hyperlipemia or as a result a defect in the glomerular basement membranes, as in Alport's syndrome. Filtered lipids accumulate in the tubular cells, tubular basement membranes and interstitial macrophages. Both the protein and the lipid overload may damage the tubular cells, which then desquamate. Desquamated cells loaded with lipid tend to calcify.

Advanced Sclerosing Glomerular Diseases

Tubulo-interstitial abnormalities are commonly seen in various types of chronic progressive glomerular damage (e.g., advanced [sclerosing] stages of chronic glomerulonephritis of any origin).

Tubular atrophy is caused mainly by ischemia due to insufficient blood flow through the contracted glomerular bed and to vascular sclerosis induced by hypertension, which accompanies the glomerular sclerosis. Possible contributing variables include progression of the direct tubular damage that had occurred in the acute or active stage of the disease, and perhaps even obliteration of renal lymphatics. Interstitial fibrosis is probably secondary to tubular atrophy and ischemia but, on occasion, severe interstitial inflammation may in itself lead to scarring. Inflammatory infiltrates that accompany tubular atrophy consist mainly of lymphocytes but also of some histiocytes. Polymorphonuclear leukocytes are occasionally seen in tubular lumina or in interstitial tissue. It is uncertain whether these leukocytes represent a reaction to active cellular degeneration of the tubules or are evidence of ascending infection promoted by decreased flow of urine.

Ischemic Atrophy

The renal parenchymal lesions that are associated with gradual occlusion of renal arteries are known as ischemic atrophy.

This condition affects tubules, interstitial tissue and glomeruli, and the extent and distribution of the parenchymal changes depend on the size and distribution of the vessels that have been occluded (see volume on Vascular Diseases).

Vascular disease is so common that pathologists have to exclude ischemic atrophy before reaching a diagnosis of tubulo-interstitial nephritis-associated fibrosis.

End-stage Kidney

End-stage kidney occurs when severe atrophy and sclerosis of an entire kidney are so advanced that it is no longer possible to determine the nature of the original disease or to establish with certainty whether it began in the glomeruli, tubulo-interstitial tissue or blood vessels. End-stage kidney was seldom seen in the past, but now it is a common finding in long-term dialysis patients.

Tubulo-interstitial changes consist of extensive tubular atrophy and interstitial fibrosis, accompanied by mild to moderate infiltration by inflammatory cells, mainly small lymphocytes. Sometimes, focal calcification and metaplastic cartilage and bone formation are found. Oxalate crystals are a common occurrence. Some tubules, instead of becoming atrophic, undergo hyperplasia and dilatation, becoming cysts of various sizes. This "acquired cystic disease" often is characterized by atypia of the lining epithelium and, on occasion, by development of a carcinoma in a cyst.

Arteries usually develop intimal thickening and luminal narrowing ("disuse endarteritis"). In addition, there is a reduction of the medial musculature and an increase in the medial ground substance and, quite often, focal nodular hyperplasia of the smooth muscle. Similar changes may be seen in the veins, which, in addition, often show thrombosis.

(Glomerular lesions—see volume on Glomerular Diseases)

Tubulo-interstitial Lesions in Glomerular and Vascular Diseases
Acute and Chronic Glomerular Diseases

Fig. 13-1 Acute interstitial inflammation in a case of diffuse proliferative glomerulonephritis. Periglomerular infiltration by histiocytes, lymphocytes, plasma cells and occasional polymorphonuclear neutrophils and eosinophils. (hematoxylin and eosin, $\times 270$)

Fig. 13-2 Tubular atrophy and interstitial fibrosis in a case of advanced sclerosing glomerulonephritis. Similar changes can be seen in ischemic atrophy of the kidney. (periodic acid-Schiff, $\times 110$)

Fig. 13-3 Proteinuria with massive cast formation and renal insufficiency in a case of lupus nephritis. (periodic acid-Schiff, $\times 110$)

End-stage Kidney

Fig. 13-4 End-stage kidney. Considerable atrophy and numerous acquired cortical cysts.

Fig. 13-5 End-stage kidney. Extensive glomerular sclerosis, tubular atrophy and dilatation, scattered hyaline casts, interstitial fibrosis and arteriosclerosis. (periodic acid-Schiff, $\times 110$)

Fig. 13-6 Same patient as in Figure 13-5. End-stage kidney, left in place more than 10 years. Almost complete disappearance of glomeruli. Tubules are extensively filled with hyaline casts ("thyroidization"). (periodic acid-Schiff, $\times 270$)

194

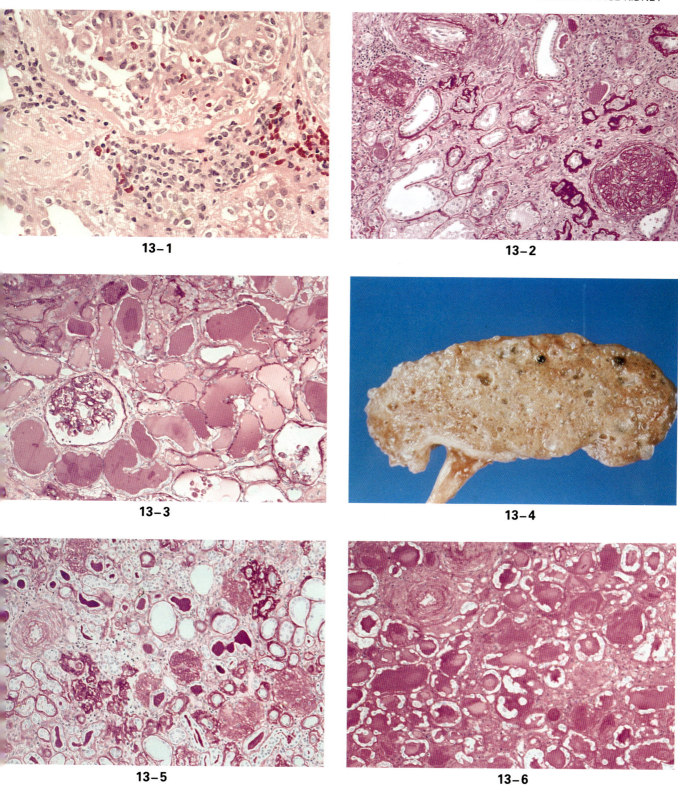

13–1

13–2

13–3

13–4

13–5

13–6

End-stage Kidney

Fig. 13-7   Another area of the kidney shown in Figure 13-6. Vascular sclerosis and interstitial fibrosis. A remnant of a glomerulus is seen near the right corner; a partly preserved tubule with clear cells is on the left. (periodic acid-Schiff, ×270)

Fig. 13-8   Histologic section from kidney shown in Figure 13-4. Numerous cysts lined by flattened, very thin epithelium. (elastic-van Gieson's stain, ×50)

Fig. 13-9   Same kidney as in Figure 13-8. Cyst lined by hyperplastic epithelium forming numerous papillae. (periodic acid-Schiff, ×270)

Fig. 13-10   Section from end-stage kidney showing tubular foam cells. Compare with Figure 13-7. (periodic acid-Schiff, ×220)

Fig. 13-11   Clusters of proliferating "embryonal cells" forming small tumor-like nodules that resemble small Wilms' tumors. (periodic acid-Schiff, ×220)

Fig. 13-12   Osteoid-like lamellae formed in cortical interstitium. (trichrome, ×220)

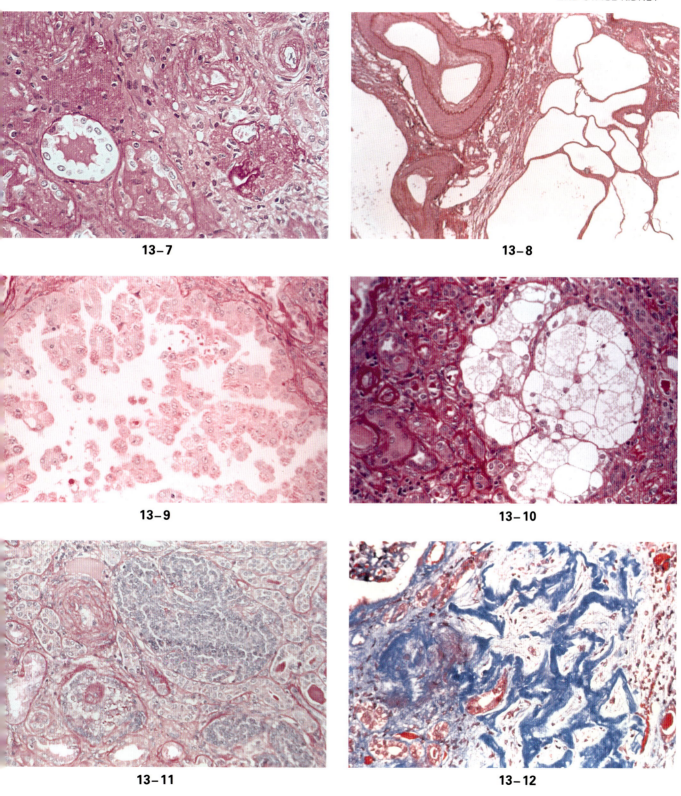

13–7

13–8

13–9

13–10

13–11

13–12

14

Miscellaneous Disorders

Miscellaneous Disorders

Radiation Nephritis

In human beings, tubular cells are quite sensitive to radiation. With moderate doses, the cells become atrophic, cuboidal or flattened and have clear cytoplasm. With large doses, frank necrosis and desquamation are evident, leaving denuded basement membrane. Regeneration often is abnormal, so that the cells have poorly formed cytoplasm and abnormal nuclei. The new cells may, in turn, degenerate and be replaced by third, fourth and subsequent generations. Each generation forms a new layer of basement membrane and, after some time, the tubules become surrounded by a thick, layered structure that resembles tree bark. The interstitium undergoes extensive fibrosis, with little evidence of inflammation. Steps in the development of these changes are best followed in the experimental model with an appropriate animal, such as the rat.

(For glomerular changes see volume on Glomerular Diseases)

(For vascular changes see volume on Vascular Diseases)

Balkan Endemic Nephropathy

This form of nephropathy is a chronic and fatal renal disease endemic to restricted areas of Yugoslavia, Rumania and Bulgaria, within the Danube Basin. It was common in the past but has become rare in recent years.

Clinical Features: The disease occurs between the ages of 30 and 60 years and is manifested by lumbar pain, intermittent hematuria, bacteriuria, rarely proteinuria, anemia and nephrolithiasis. The onset is insidious, and renal insufficiency is progressive: 50% of patients succumb within two years of diagnosis; the rest die within 10 years. The disease affects mainly the farming population. The urine contains increased amounts of β-microglobulin.

There is a 30% to 40% incidence of benign and malignant transitional cell tumors of the urinary tract.

The geographic distribution seems to indicate exposure to environmental agents. Trace elements (cadmium, uranium, lead, silicon, environmental radioactivity) or bacterial agents (leptospira, brucella, coliforms and streptococci) have not been detected. Nephrotoxins of plant origin or fungi, especially *Penicillium verrucosum* var. *cyclopium* and ochratoxin A, have been found to produce renal lesions similar to Balkan endemic nephropathy in rats and pigs. Slow porcine coronaviruses have been suspected as a possible cause. To date, the offending agent or agents have not been identified with certainty.

Macroscopic Findings: In the later stages of the disease, the kidneys are bilaterally and symmetrically small and smooth, with finely granular cortical surfaces. They usually weigh between 20 and 60 g.

Light Microscopic Findings: In the early stages, there is degeneration of tubular epithelium, focal atrophy of tubules and interstitial edema and fibrosis, with mild lymphocytic interstitial infiltrates. Later lesions show widespread and extensive loss of tubules and interstitial fibrosis, with variable, generally small, numbers of chronic inflammatory cells. Glomerular sclerosis and hyalinization may be found in subcapsular areas, where the disease is most severe. Vascular lesions usually are mild.

Electron Microscopic Findings: Changes visualized by electron microscopy are nonspecific, although osmiophilic bodies (0.1 to 0.5 μm in diameter) have been found in tubular epithelial cytoplasm.

Granulomatous Sarcoid Nephropathy

This term refers to widespread involvement of the renal parenchyma by sarcoid granulomas with development of renal insufficiency.

Clinical Features: Sarcoid lesions in the kidneys as incidental findings are found frequently (7% to 19% of cases) at autopsy in cases of generalized sarcoidosis but have little clinical relevance. Impairment of renal function in sarcoidosis may be attributed to hypercalcemia, due to enhanced calcium absorption from the gut, with nephrocalcinosis and renal calculi. Renal insufficiency as a result of direct involvement of the renal parenchyma by the granulomatous process occurs in approximately 2% of cases and is reversible with corticosteroid therapy.

The causative agent or agents have not been identified, and the granulomatous reaction is believed to represent an immunologic hypersensitivity to widely disseminated antigens that either have a low solubility or that cannot be metabolized. The Kveim test is positive, and the tuberculin test is negative.

Macroscopic Findings: With extensive infiltration the kidneys are enlarged. In the "healing" stages, the kidneys are fibrotic and contracted.

Microscopic Findings: The interstitium shows noncaseating granulomas composed of epithelioid cells and giant cells, with a lymphocytic border and loose connective tissue. Schaumann's and asteroid bodies are rare.

The healing lesions lead to dense interstitial fibrosis, tubular atrophy and focal thickening of tubular basement membranes. Focal areas of calcium deposition may be found in the medulla. Arterioles show intimal thickening and hyaline deposits. Because of its focal nature the disease may be missed in a needle biopsy specimen.

A variable glomerular morphologic picture of mesangial cell proliferation, endocapillary proliferation and sclerosing and membranous lesions can occur. Immunofluorescence studies demonstrate glomerular deposits of IgG.

Tubulo-interstitial Nephritis of Unknown Etiologic Basis (idiopathic)

This category includes tubulo-interstitial nephritides that are not related to renal infection or drug administration and whose causes are unknown.

Acute Idiopathic Tubulo-interstitial Nephritis

Acute eosinophilic tubulo-interstitial nephritis and renal failure, with bone marrow-lymph node granulomas and anterior uveitis, has been reported. Patients showed hypergammaglobulinemia and had an elevated erythrocyte sedimentation rate. Presenting symptoms included flank pain, abdominal cramps, nausea and malaise. The process resolved over two years. No etiologic agent was found, but it is possible that damage within the renal parenchyma stimulated an eosinophilic and mononuclear response, with concomitant lymphohistiocytic activation and granuloma formation in lymph nodes and bone marrow.

Histologic studies showed focal tubular necrosis and interstitial infiltration by lymphocytes, plasma cells and eosinophils. No granulomas were seen in the kidneys, but they occurred in bone marrow and lymph nodes.

Fluorescence microscopy revealed no abnormality.

Idiopathic Granulomatous Tubulo-interstitial Nephritis

Granulomas occasionally are found in cases that are not due to tuberculosis, sarcoid, actinomycetes, aspergilli, toxoplasma, drug administration or other agents known to evoke a granulomatous response. The above term is used in these cases unless the etiologic basis and pathogenetic features are known.

Chronic Idiopathic Tubulo-interstitial Nephritis

There are a small number of cases of focal or diffuse chronic tubulo-interstitial nephritis with or without pelvic scarring in which the etiologic basis is unknown. Chronic pyelonephritis associated with obstruction, vesicoureteral reflux or analgesic nephropathy has been excluded. The term *chronic idiopathic tubulo-interstitial nephritis* is used unless the etiologic basis and pathogenetic features have been determined.

201

Miscellaneous Disorders
Radiation Nephritis

Fig. 14-1   Chronic radiation nephritis in a child. Patient was treated for hepatoma, and the kidney was included in the field of radiation. Extensive sclerosis of glomeruli, diffuse tubular atrophy and mild inflammatory infiltration. (hematoxylin and eosin, ×45)

Fig. 14-2   Same case as in Figure 14-1. Tubular atrophy and interstitial fibrosis. Some dilated tubules show desquamation of cells and fragments of casts that are slightly stained with bile. (hematoxylin and eosin, ×270)

Fig. 14-3   Experimental radiation nephritis. Kidney three and one-half months after administration of 4800 rads to a rat. Tubular atrophy and regeneration with many atypical cells. (hematoxylin and eosin, ×430)

Balkan Endemic Nephropathy

Fig. 14-4   Balkan nephropathy. Extensive tubular atrophy, interstitial fibrosis and scanty lymphocytic infiltration. (hematoxylin and eosin, ×400)

Fig. 14-5   Balkan nephropathy. Papillary transitional cell carcinoma in a renal pelvis. (hematoxylin and eosin, ×135)

Sarcoidosis

Fig. 14-6   A known case of sarcoidosis with hypercalcemia, slight proteinuria and elevated blood level of urea. Noncaseous sarcoid granuloma in the renal interstitium. (hematoxylin and eosin, ×160)

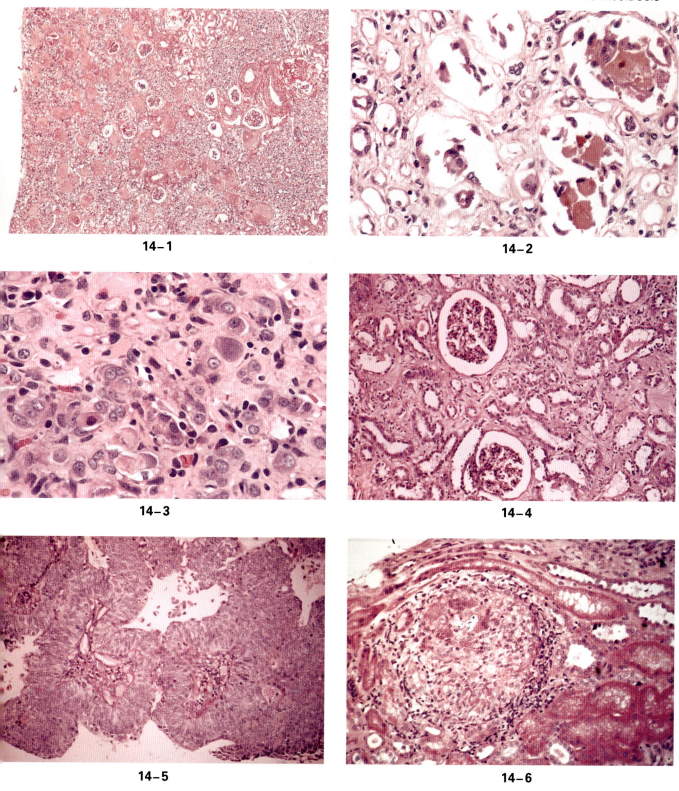

14-1

14-2

14-3

14-4

14-5

14-6

Sarcoidosis

Fig. 14-7   Another case of sarcoidosis with hypercalcemia, showing sarcoid granuloma with giant cells, tubular atrophy, interstitial fibrosis and scattered lymphocytes. (periodic acid-Schiff, ×220)

Tubulo-interstitial Nephritis of Unknown Etiologic Basis (idiopathic)
Acute Idiopathic Eosinophilic Tubulo-interstitial Nephritis

Fig. 14-8   Diffuse interstitial inflammation of a kidney with many eosinophils. (hematoxylin and eosin, ×430)

Fig. 14-9   Sister of the patient illustrated in Figure 14-8. Similar interstitial inflammation with many eosinophils. (hematoxylin and eosin, ×1100)

Idiopathic Granulomatous Tubulo-interstitial Nephritis

Fig. 14-10   Granulomatous interstitial nephritis with chronic renal failure. A 23-year-old man with a history of alcoholism, allergy and "granulomatous" hepatitis. Diffuse interstitial inflammation, peritubular granuloma and destruction of tubules (hematoxylin and eosin, ×160).

Fig. 14-11   Another area from the case shown in Figure 14-10 showing multinucleated giant cells. (periodic acid-Schiff, ×160)

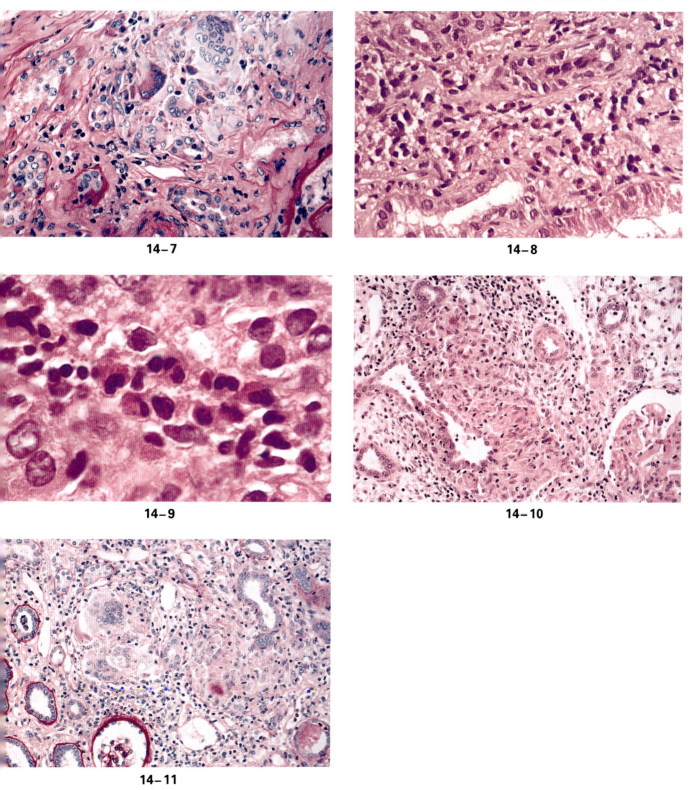

14–7

14–8

14–9

14–10

14–11

Radiation Nephritis

Fig. 14-12 Experimental radiation nephritis in a rat. Tubule in the center shows marked thickening, "splitting" and wrinkling of its basement membrane. Tubule on the left shows less striking changes, consisting mainly of splitting or reduplication of basement membrane. (electron micrograph, ×5200)

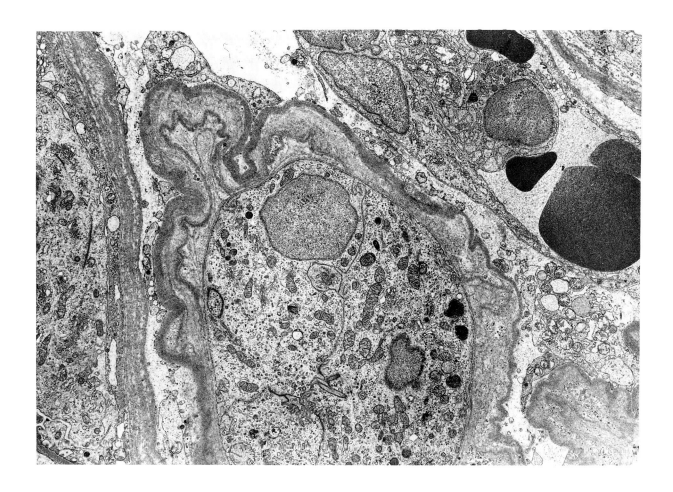

REFERENCES

Included in this list are books dealing with renal pathology and books dealing with clinical nephrology. Most books in the latter category have good sections on renal pathology and normal histology.

Asscher, A.W., Moffat, D.B., and Sander, E.: *Nephrology Illustrated*. Philadelphia: W.B. Saunders, 1982.

Becker, E.L. (Ed.): *Structural Basis of Renal Disease*. New York: Hoeber Medical Division, 1968.

Black, D.A.K., and Jones, N.F. (Eds.): *Renal Disease* (4th edition). Oxford: Blackwell Scientific Publications, 1979.

Brenner, B.M., and Rector, F.C., Jr. (Eds.): *The Kidney* (2nd edition). Philadelphia: W.B. Saunders, 1981.

Brun, C., and Olsen, S.: *Atlas of Renal Biopsy* Copenhagen: Munksgaard, 1980.

Churg, J., and Sobin, L.H.: *Renal Disease: Classification and Atlas of Glomerular Diseases*. Tokyo and New York: Igaku-Shoin, 1982.

Churg, J., Spargo, B.H., Mostofi, F.K., et al. (Eds.): *Kidney Disease: Present Status*. Baltimore: Williams & Wilkins, 1979.

Cotran, R.S., Brenner, B.M., and Stein, J.H. (Eds.): *Tubulo-Interstitial Nephropathies*. New York: Churchill Livingstone, 1983.

Darmady, E.M., and MacIver, A.G.: *Renal Pathology*. London and Boston: Butterworths, 1980.

Earley, L.E., and Gottschalk, C.W. (Eds.): *Strauss and Welt's Diseases of the Kidney* (3rd edition). Boston: Little, Brown, 1979.

Edelmann, C.M. (Ed.): *Pediatric Kidney Disease*. Boston: Little, Brown, 1978.

Elkin, M.: *Radiology of the Urinary System*. Boston: Little, Brown, 1980.

Hamburger, J., Crosnier, J., and Grunfeld, J.P. (Eds.): *Nephrology*. New York: John Wiley & Sons (Paris: Flammarion Medecine-Sciences [French edition]), 1979.

Heptinstall, R.H.: *Pathology of the Kidney* (3rd edition). Boston: Little, Brown, 1983.

International Committee for Nomenclature and Nosology of Renal Disease: *A Handbook of Kidney Nomenclature and Nosology*. Boston: Little, Brown, 1975.

Kincaid-Smith, P.: *The Kidney*. Oxford: Blackwell Scientific Publications, 1975.

Kuhn, K., and Brod, J.: *Contributions to Nephrology*. Volume 16: *Interstitial Nephropathies*. Basel: S. Karger, 1979.

Massry, S.G., and Glassock, R.J.: *Textbook of Nephrology*. Baltimore and London: Williams & Wilkins, 1983.

Meadows, R.: *Renal Histopathology* (2nd edition). Oxford: Oxford University Press, 1978.

Risdon, R.A., and Turner, D.R.: *Atlas of Renal Pathology*. Philadelphia and Toronto: J.B. Lippincott, 1980.

Royer, P., Habib, R., Mathieu, H., et al.: *Pediatric Nephrology*. Philadelphia: W.B. Saunders, 1973.

Solez, K., and Whelton, A. (Eds.): *Acute Renal Failure*. New York: Marcel Dekker, 1983.

Spargo, B.H., Seymour, A.E., and Ordonez, N.: *Renal Biopsy Pathology*. New York: John Wiley & Sons, 1980.

Zollinger, H.U., and Mihatsch, M.J.: *Renal Pathology in Biopsy*. Berlin, Heidelberg and New York: Springer-Verlag, 1978.

Chapter 1

Cogan, M.G.: Tubulo-interstitial nephropathies: A pathophysiologic approach. Medical staff conference, University of California, San Francisco. *West. J. Med.* 132:134, 1980.

Cogan, M.G.: Classification and patterns of renal dysfunction. In Cotran, R.S., Brenner, B.M., and Stein, J.H. (Eds.): *Tubulo-Interstitial Nephritis*. New York, Edinburgh, London and Melbourne: Churchill Livingstone, 1983, pp. 35–48.

Cotran, R.S.: Interstitial nephritis. In Churg, J., Spargo, B.H., Mostofi, F.K., et al. (Eds.): *Kidney Disease: Present Status*. Baltimore: Williams & Wilkins, 1979, pp. 254–280.

Cotran, R.S.: Tubulointerstitial diseases. In Brenner, B.M., and Rector, F.C., Jr. (Eds.): *The Kidney* (2nd edition). Philadelphia: W.B. Saunders, 1981, pp. 1633–1667.

Chapter 2

Bohman, S.O.: The ultrastructure of the renal interstitium. In Cotran, R.S., Brenner, B.M., and Stein, J.H. (Eds.): *Tubulo-Interstitial Nephropathies*. New York, Edinburgh, London and Melbourne: Churchill Livingstone, 1983, pp. 1–34.

Bulger, R.E.: Kidney morphology. In Earley, L.E., and Gottschalk, C.W. (Eds.): *Strauss and Welt's Diseases of the Kidney* (3rd edition). Boston: Little, Brown, 1979, pp. 3–39.

Bulger, R.E., and Nagle, R.B.: Ultrastructure of the interstitium in the rabbit kidney. *Amer. J. Anat.* 136:183, 1973.

Chapman, W.H., Bulger, R.E., Cutler, R.E., et al.: *The Urinary System*. Philadelphia: W.B. Saunders, 1973.

Jones, D.B.: Scanning electron microscopy of isolated dog renal tubules. *Scanning Electron Microsc.* II:805, 1982.

Maunsbach, A.B., Olsen, S.T., and Christensen, E.I. (Eds.): *Functional Ultrastructure of the Kidney* London: Academic Press, 1980.

Tisher, C.C.: Anatomy of the kidney. In Brenner, B.M., and Rector, F.C. (Eds.): *The Kidney* (2nd edition). Philadelphia: W.B. Saunders, 1976, pp. 3–64.

REFERENCES

Chapter 3

Bengtsson, U: Long-term pattern in chronic pyelonephritis. *Contrib. Nephrol.* 16:31, 1979.

Cotran, R.S., and Pennington, J.E.: Urinary tract infection, pyelonephritis, and reflux nephropathy. In Brenner, B.M., and Rector, F.C., Jr. (Eds.): *The Kidney* (2nd edition). Philadelphia: W.B. Saunders, 1981, pp. 1571–1632.

Gillenwater, J.W., Harrison, R.B., and Kunin, C.M.: Natural history of bacteriuria in schoolgirls: A long-term case control study. *N. Engl. J. Med.* 301:396, 1979.

Holland, N.H., Kotchen, T., and Bhathena, D.: Hypertension in children with chronic pyelonephritis. *Kidney Int.* 8:S–243, 1975.

Kass, E.H., and Brumfitt, W. (Eds.): *Infections of the Urinary Tract.* Chicago: University of Chicago Press, 1978.

Kincaid Smith, P., and Fairley, K.F. (Eds.): *Renal Infection and Renal Scarring.* Melbourne: Mercedes, 1970.

Losse, H., Asscher, A.W., and Lison, A.E. (Eds.): *Pyelonephritis.* Volume 4: *Urinary Tract Infections.* Stuttgart and New York: Georg Heime Verlag, 1980.

Miller, T., and Phillips, S.: Pyelonephritis: The relationship between infection, renal scarring, and antimicrobial therapy. *Kidney Int.* 19:654, 1981.

Murray, T., and Goldberg, J.: Chronic interstitial nephritis: Etiologic factors. *Ann. Intern. Med.* 82:453, 1975.

Pasternack, A., Helin, H., Vantlinen, T., et al.: Acute tubulointerstitial nephritis in a patient with Mycoplasma pneumoniae infection. *Scand. J. Infect. Dis.* 11:85, 1979.

Paulter, N., Gabriel, R., Porter, K.A., et al.: Acute interstitial nephritis complicating Legionnaire's disease. *Clin. Nephrol.* 15:216, 1981.

Rosen, S., Harmon, W., Krensky, A.M., et al.: Tubulo-interstitial nephritis associated with polyomavirus (BK type) infection. *N. Engl. J. Med.* 308:1192, 1983.

Smellie, J.M., Normand, I.C.S., and Katz, G.: Children with urinary infection: A comparison of those with and those without vesicoureteric reflux. *Kidney Int.* 20:717, 1981.

Svanborg Eden, C., Hagberg, L., Hanson, L.A., et al.: Bacterial adherence and urinary tract infection. *Lancet* 1:961, 1982.

Chapter 4

Abdou, N.I., NaPombejara, C., Sagawa, A., et al.: Malakoplakia: Evidence for monocyte lysosomal abnormality correctable by cholinergic agonist in vitro and in vivo. *N. Engl. J. Med.* 297:1413, 1977.

Cadnapaphornchai, P., Rosenberg, B.F., Taher, S., et al.: Renal parenchymal malakoplakia: An unusual cause of renal failure. *N. Engl. J. Med.* 299:1110, 1978.

Case Records of the Massachusetts General Hospital: Granulomatous interstitial nephritis in leprosy. *N. Engl. J. Med.* 300:546, 1979.

Damjanov, I., and Katz, S.M.: Malakoplakia. *Pathol. Annu.* 16(2):103, 1981.

Goodman, M., Curry, T., and Russell, T.: Xanthogranulomatous pyelonephritis (XGP): A local disease with sys-

temic manifestations: Report of 23 patients and review of the literature. *Medicine (Baltimore)* 58:171, 1979.

Jander, H.P., Pujara, S., and Murad, T.M.: Tumefactive megalocytic interstitial nephritis. *Radiology* 129:635, 1978.

Malek, R.S., and Elder, J.S.: Xanthogranulomatous pyelonephritis: A critical analysis of 26 cases and of the literature. *J. Urol.* 119:589, 1978.

Rich, A.R.: The pathology of 19 cases of a peculiar and special form of nephritis associated with acquired syphilis. *Bull. Johns Hopkins Hosp.* 50:357, 1932.

Steer, A.: Pathogenesis of renal changes in epidemic hemorrhagic fever. In Mostofi, F.K., and Smith, D.E. (Eds.): *The Kidney.* Baltimore: Williams and Wilkins, 1966, pp. 476–487.

Chapter 5

Acute Disease

Appel, G.B.: A decade of penicillin-related acute interstitial nephritis—more questions than answers. *Clin. Nephrol.* 13:151, 1980.

Bennett, W.M.: Aminoglycoside nephrotoxicity. *Nephron* 35:73, 1983.

Dixon, A.J., Winearls, C.G., and Dunhill, M.S.: Interstitial nephritis. *J. Clin. Pathol.* 34:616, 1981.

Ellis, D., Fried, W.A., Yunis, E.J., et al.: Acute interstitial nephritis in children: A report of 13 cases and review of the literature. *Pediatrics* 67:862, 1981.

Fialk, M.A., Romankiewicz, J., Perrone, F., et al.: Allergic interstitial nephritis with diuretics. *Ann. Intern. Med.* 81:403, 1974.

Grussendorf, M., Andrassy, K., Waldherr, R., et al.: Systemic hypersensitivity to allopurinol with acute interstitial nephritis. *Amer. J. Nephrol.* 1:105, 1981.

Hale, D.H.: Interstitial nephritis and cimetidine. *Ann. Intern. Med.* 94:416, 1981.

Houghton, D.C., Campbell-Boswell, M.V., Bennett, W.M., et al.: Myeloid bodies in the renal tubules of humans: Relationship to gentamicin therapy. *Clin. Nephrol.* 10:140, 1978.

Linton, A.L., Clark, W.F., Drieger, A.A., et al.: Acute interstitial nephritis due to drugs. *Ann. Intern. Med.* 93:735, 1980.

Saltissi, D., Pusey, C.D., and Rainford, D.J.: Recurrent acute renal failure due to antibiotic-induced interstitial nephritis. *Brit. Med. J.* 1:1182, 1979.

Sigala, J.F., Biava, G.G., and Hulter, H.N.: Red blood cell casts in acute interstitial nephritis. *Arch. Intern. Med.* 138:1419, 1978.

Wood, B.C., Sharma, J.N., Germann, D.R., et al.: Gallium citrate Ga67 imaging in noninfectious interstitial nephritis. *Arch. Intern. Med.* 138:1665, 1978.

Chronic Disease

Aurell, M., Svalander, C., Wallin, L., et al.: Renal function and biopsy findings in patients on long-term lithium treatment. *Kidney Int.* 20:663, 1981.

Axelson, R.A.: Analgesic induced renal papillary necrosis in the Gunn rat: The comparative nephrotoxicity of aspirin and phenacetin. *J. Pathol.* 120:145, 1976.

Blohmé, I., and Johansson, S.: Renal pelvic neoplasms and atypical urothelium in patients with end-stage analgesic nephropathy. *Kidney Int.* 20:671, 1981.

Gloor, F.: Changing concepts in pathogenesis and morphology of analgesic nephropathy as seen in Europe. *Kidney Int.* 13:27, 1978.

Hare, W., and Poynter, J.D.: The radiology of renal papillary necrosis as seen in analgesic nephropathy. *Clin. Radiol.* 25:423, 1974.

Harmon, W.E., Cohen, H.J., Schnuberger, E.E., et al.: Chronic renal failure in children treated with methyl-CCNU. *N. Engl. J. Med.* 300:1200, 1979.

Hestbech, J., Hansen, H.E., Amdisen, A., et al.: Chronic renal lesions following long-term treatment with lithium. *Kidney Int.* 12:205, 1977.

Kling, M.A., Fox, J.G., Johnston, S.M., Talkoff-Rubin, N.E., Rubin, R.H., and Calvin, R.B.: Effects of long-term lithium administration on renal structure and function in rats. *Lab. Invest.* 50:526, 1984.

Mihatsch, M.J., Torhorst, J., Steinmann, E., et al.: The morphologic diagnosis of analgesic (phenacetin) abuse. *Pathol. Res. Pract.* 164:68, 1979.

Murray, T., and Goldberg, M.: Analgesic-associated nephropathy in the U.S.A.: Epidemiologic, clinical and pathogenetic features. *Kidney Int.* 13:64, 1978.

Singer, I.: Lithium and the kidney. *Kidney Int.* 19:374, 1981.

Chapter 6

Andres, G., Albini, B., and Ossi, E.: Pathogenesis, diagnosis, prognosis and treatment of immunologically mediated tubulointerstitial nephritides. In Coggins, C.H., and Cummings, N.B. (Eds.): *Prevention of Kidney and Urinary Tract Diseases* (DHEW Publ. No. [NIH] 78–855). Washington, D.C.: U.S. Department of Health, Education and Welfare, 1978, pp. 251–262.

Andres, G.A., and McCluskey, R.T.: Tubular and interstitial renal diseases due to immunological mechanisms. *Kidney Int.* 7:271, 1975.

Baldamus, C.A., Kachel, G., Koch, C., et al.: Cellular immune mechanisms in experimental tubulointerstitial nephritis (TIN). *Contrib. Nephrol.* 16:141, 1979.

Bergstein, J., and Lifman, N.: Interstitial nephritis with anti-tubular-basement-membrane antibody. *N. Engl. J. Med.* 292:875, 1975.

Border, W.A., Lehman, D.H., Egan, J.D., et al.: Anti-tubular basement membrane antibodies in methicillin-associated interstitial nephritis. *N. Engl. J. Med.* 291:381, 1974.

Brentjens, J.R., Noble, B., and Andres, G.A.: Immunologically mediated lesions of kidney tubules and interstitium in laboratory animals and in man. In Wilson, C., Miescher, P.A., and Mueller-Eberhard, H.J. (Eds.): *Renal Immunopathology.* New York: Springer Verlag: 1982, pp. 357–378.

Cotran, R.S., and Galvanek, E.: Immunopathology of human tubulointerstitial diseases: Localization of immunoglobulins, complement and Tamm-Horsfall protein. *Contrib. Nephrol.* 16:126, 1979.

Hyman, L.R., Ballow, M., and Kniesser, M.R.: Diphenylhydantoin interstitial nephritis: Roles of cellular and humoral immunologic injury. *J. Pediatr.* 92:915, 1978.

Hyun, J., and Galen, M.A.: Acute interstitial nephritis. A case characterized by increase in serum IgG, IgM, and IgE concentrations, eosinophilia and IgE deposition in renal tubules. *Arch. Intern. Med.* 141:679, 1981.

McCluskey, R.T., and Bhan, A.K.: Cell-mediated mechanisms in renal diseases. *Kidney Int.* 21(Suppl. 11):S–6, 1982.

McCluskey, R.T., and Colvin, R.G.: Immunological aspects of renal tubular and interstitial diseases. *Annu. Rev. Med.* 29:191, 1978.

Moorthy, A.V., and Pringle, D.: Urticaria, vasculitis, hypocomplementemia, and immune-complex glomerulonephritis. *Arch. Pathol. Lab. Med.* 106:68, 1982.

Ooi, B.S., Ooi, Y.M., Mohini, R., et al.: Humoral mechanisms in drug induced acute interstitial nephritis. *Clin. Immunol. Immunopathol.* 10:330, 1978.

Orfila, C., Rakotoarivony, J., Durand, D., et al.: A correlative study of immunofluorescence, electron, and light microscopy in immunologically mediated renal tubular disease in man. *Nephron* 23:14, 1979.

Watson, A.J.S., Dalbow, M.H., Stachura, I., et al.: Immunologic studies in cimetidine-induced nephropathy and polymyositis. *N. Engl. J. Med.* 308:142, 1983.

Winer, R.L., Cohen, A.H., Sawhney, A.S., et al.: Sjogren's syndrome with immune complex tubulointerstitial renal disease. *Clin. Immunol. Immunopathol.* 8:494, 1977.

Chapter 7

Cotran, R.S.: Glomerulosclerosis in reflux nephropathy. *Kidney Int.* 21:528, 1982.

Fasth, A., Ahlstedt, S., Hanson, L.A., et al.: Cross reaction between Tamm-Horsfall glycoprotein and Escherichia coli. *Int. Arch. Allergy Appl. Immunol.* 63:303, 1980.

Habib, R.: Pathology of renal segmental corticopapillary scarring in children with hypertension: The concept of segmental hypoplasia. In Hodson, C.J., and Kincaid-Smith, P. (Eds.): *Reflux Nephropathy.* New York: Masson Publishing, 1979, pp. 220–239.

Heale, W.F., and Ferguson, R.S.: The pathogenesis of renal scarring in children. In Brumfitt, W., and Kass, E.H. (Eds.): *Urinary Tract Infections.* Chicago: University of Chicago Press, 1979.

Hodson, C.J., and Kincaid-Smith, P. (Eds.): *Reflux Nephropathy.* New York: Masson Publishing, 1979.

Hodson, C.J.: The diffuse form of reflux nephropathy in urinary tract infection. In Losse, H., Asscher, W., and Lison, A. (Eds.): *Pyelonephritis.* Stuttgart and New York: Georg Heime Verlag, 1980, vol. 4, pp. 84–90.

Hodson, C.J., Heptinstall, R.H., and Winberg, J. (Eds.): Contributions to Nephrology. Volume 39: *Reflux Nephropathy Update: 1983.* Basel: S. Karger, 1984.

REFERENCES

Klahr, S., Buerkert, J., and Purkerson, M.: The kidney in obstructive uropathy. *Contrib. Nephrol.* 7:220, 1977.

McCurdy, F.A., and Vernier, R.L.: Unique consequences of kidney infections in infants and children: Pathogenesis, early recognition and prevention of scarring. *Amer. J. Nephrol.* 1:184, 1981.

Ransley, P.G.: The renal papilla, intrarenal reflux and chronic pyelonephritis. In Zurukzoglu, W., Papidimitrion, M., Pyrpasopoulos, M. et al.: (Eds.): *Advances in Basic and Clinical Nephrology.* Basel: S. Karger, 1981, pp. 363–367.

Ransley, P.G., and Risdon, R.A.: The pathogenesis of reflux nephropathy. *Brit. J. Radiol.* 14(Supplement):1, 1978.

Shah, K.J., Robins, D.G., and White, R.H.R.: Renal scarring and vesicoureteric reflux. *Arch. Dis. Child.* 53:210, 1978.

Shindo, S., Bernstein, J., and Arant, B.S., Jr.: Evolution of renal segmental atrophy (Ask-Upmark kidney) in children with vesicoureteric reflux: Radiographic and morphologic studies. *J. Pediatr.* 102:847, 1983.

Smellie, J.M., Normand, I.C.M., and Katz, G.: Children with urinary infection: A comparison of those with and without VUR. *Kidney Int.* 20:717, 1981.

Solez, K., and Heptinstall, B.H.: Intra-renal urinary extravasation with formation of venous polyps containing Tamm-Horsfall protein. *J. Urol.* 119:180, 1977.

Torres, V.E., Velosa, J.A., Holley, K.E., et al.: The progression of vesicoureteral reflux nephropathy. *Ann. Intern. Med.* 92:776, 1980.

Zager, R.A., Cotran, R.S., and Hoyer, J.R.: Pathologic localization of Tamm-Horsfall protein in interstitial deposits in renal disease. *Lab. Invest.* 38:52, 1978.

Chapter 8

Alleyne, G.A.O., Van Eps, L.W.S., and Addae, S.: The kidney in sickle cell anemia. *Kidney Int.* 7:371, 1975.

Chrisprin, A.R., Hull, D., Lillie, J.G., et al.: Renal tubular necrosis and papillary necrosis after gastroenteritis in infants. *Brit. Med. J.* 1:410, 1970.

Davies, D.J., Kennedy A., and Roberts, C.: Renal medullary necrosis in infancy and childhood. *J. Pathol.* 99:125, 1969.

Eknoyan, G., Qunibi, W.Y., Grissom, R.T., et al.: Renal papillary necrosis: An update. *Medicine (Baltimore)* 61:55, 1982.

Gloor, F.: Uber verschiedene Formen der Papillennekrosen der Nieren. *Pathol. Microbiol.* 23:263, 1960.

Jennette, J.C., Sheps, D.S., and McNeill, D.D.: Exclusively vascular systemic amyloidosis with visceral ischemia. *Arch. Pathol. Lab. Med.* 106:323, 1982.

Lindvall, N.: Radiological changes of renal papillary necrosis. *Kidney Int.* 13:93, 1978.

Sabatini, S., Koppera, S., Manaligod, J., et al.: Role of urinary concentrating ability in the generation of toxic papillary necrosis. *Kidney Int.* 23:705, 1983.

Watanabe, T., Nagafuchi, Y., Yoshikawa, Y., et al.: Renal papillary necrosis associated with Wegener's granulomatosis. *Hum. Pathol.* 14:551, 1983.

Chapter 9

Berndt, W.O., and Nechay, B.R.: Symposium: Toxic effects of metals on the kidney and cardiovascular system. *Fed. Proc. Fed. Amer. Soc. Exp. Biol.* 42:2955, 1983.

Choie, D.D., Longnecker, D.S., and DelCampo, A.A.: Acute and chronic cisplatin nephrotoxicity in rats. *Lab. Invest.* 44:297, 1981.

Cramer, C.R., Hagler, H.K., Silva, F.G., et al.: Chronic interstitial nephritis associated with gold therapy. *Arch. Pathol. Lab. Med.* 107:258, 1983.

Friedman, A., and Lavtin, E.: Cis-platinum(II) diammine dichloride: Another cause of bilateral small kidney. *Urology* 15:584, 1980.

Gonzalez-Vitale, J.C., Hayes, D.M., Cvitkovic, E., et al.: The renal pathology in clinical trials of cis-platinum(II) diamminedichloride. *Cancer* 39:1362, 1977.

Goyer, R.A.: Effect of toxic, chemical and environmental factors on the kidney. In Churg, J., Spargo, B.H., Mostofi, F.K., et al. (Eds.): *Kidney Disease: Present Status.* Baltimore: Williams & Wilkins, 1979, pp. 202–217.

Goyer, R.A., and Wilson, M.H.: Lead-induced inclusion bodies. Results of ethylenediaminetetraacetic acid treatment. *Lab. Invest.* 32:149, 1975.

Hong, C.D., Hanenson, I.B., Lerner, S., et al.: Occupational exposure to lead: Effects on renal function. *Kidney Int.* 18:489, 1980.

Kazantis, G.: Cadmium nephropathy. *Contrib. Nephrol.* 16:161, 1979.

Müller, H-A. and Ramin, D.V.: Morphologie und Morphogenese der durch Schwarmetalle (Pb, Bi) hervorgerufenen Kereinschlüsse in den Hauptstück-epithelien der Rattniere, *Beitr. path. Anat.* 128:445, 1963.

Wedeen, R.P., Malik, D.K., and Batuman, V.: Detection and treatment of occupational lead nephropathy. *Arch. Intern. Med.* 139:53, 1979.

Chapter 10

Adams, P.L., Adams, F.F., Bell, P.D., et al: Impaired renal blood flow autoregulation in ischemic acute renal failure. *Kidney Int.* 18:68, 1980.

Byrd, L., and Sherman, R.L.: Radiocontrast-induced acute renal failure. *Medicine (Baltimore)* 58:270, 1979.

Cronin, R.E.: Acute renal failure with radiographic contrast media. In Knochel, J.P. (Ed.): *Seminars in Nephrology.* Volume I: *Acute Renal Failure.* New York: Longman, 1981, pp. 51–55.

Dobyan, D.C., Nagle, R.B., and Bulger, R.E.: Acute tubular necrosis in the rat kidney following sustained hypotension. *Lab. Invest.* 37:411, 1977.

Flamenbaum, W.: Pathophysiology of acute renal failure. In Solez, K., and Whelton, A. (Eds.): *Acute Renal Failure: Correlations Between Morphology and Function.* New York: Marcel Dekker, 1984, pp. 149–156.

Jones, D.B.: Ultrastructure of human acute renal failure. *Lab. Invest.* 46:254, 1982.

Mason, J., and Thiel, G. (Eds.): Workshop on the role of

medullary circulation in the pathogenesis of acute renal failure. *Nephron* 31:289, 1982.

Matthys, E., Patton, M.K., Osgood, R.W., et al.: Alterations in vascular function and morphology in acute ischemic renal failure. *Kidney Int.* 23:717, 1983.

Olsen, S.: Renal histopathology in various forms of acute anuria in man. *Kidney Int.* 10:S–2, 1976.

Solez, K.: Pathogenesis of experimental acute renal failure. *Int. Rev. Exp. Pathol.* 24:277, 1983.

Solez, K., Morel-Maroger, L., and Sraer, J.-D.: The morphology of "acute tubular necrosis" in man: Analysis of 57 renal biopsies and a comparison with the glycerol model. *Medicine (Baltimore)* 58:362, 1979.

Van Zee, B.E., Hoy, W.E., Talley, T.E., et al.: Renal injury associated with intravenous pyelography in nondiabetic and diabetic patients. *Ann. Intern. Med.* 89:51, 1978.

Venkatachalam, M.A.: Pathology of acute renal failure. In Brenner, B.B., and Stein, J.M. (Eds.): *Contemporary Issues in Nephrology. Volume 6: Acute Renal Failure.* New York: Churchill Livingstone, 1980, pp. 79–107.

Chapter 11

Batuman, V., Maesaka, J.K., Haddad, B., et al.: The role of lead in gout nephropathy. *N. Engl. J. Med.* 304:520, 1981.

Benabe, J.E., and Martinez-Maldonado, M.: Hypercalcemic nephropathy. *Arch. Intern. Med.* 138:777, 1978.

Churg, J., Spargo, B.H., Sakaguchi, H., et al.: Diagnostic electron microscopy of renal diseases. In Trump, B.F., and Jones, R.T. (Eds.): *Diagnostic Electron Microscopy.* New York: John Wiley & Sons, 1980, vol. 3, pp. 203–314.

Conger, J.D.: Acute uric acid nephropathy. *Semin. Nephrol.* 1:69, 1981.

Duffy, J.L., Suzuki, Y., and Churg, J.: Acute calcium nephropathy. *Arch. Pathol.* 91:340, 1971.

Frascino, J.A., Vanamee, P., and Rosen, P.P.: Renal oxalosis and azotemia after methoxyflurane anesthesia. *N. Engl. J. Med.* 283:676, 1970.

Hodgkinson, A.: *Oxalic Acid in Biology and Medicine.* New York: Academic Press, 1977.

Klinenberg, J.R., Kippen, I., and Bluestone, R.: Hyperuricemic nephropathy: Pathologic features and factors influencing urate deposition. *Nephron* 14:88, 1975.

Salyer, W.R., and Keren, D.: Oxalosis as a complication of chronic renal failure. *Kidney Int.* 4:61, 1973.

Spargo, B.H.: Renal changes with potassium depletion. In Becker, E.L. (Ed.): *Structural Basis of Renal Disease.* New York: Harper & Row, 1968, pp. 565–586.

Yu, T.-F., and Berger, L. (Eds.). *The Kidney in Gout and Hyperuricemia.* New York: Futura Publishing, 1982.

Chapter 12

Clyne, D.H., Pesce, A.J., Thompson, R.E., et al.: Nephrotoxicity of Bence Jones proteins in the rat: Impor-

tance of protein isoelectric point. *Kidney Int.* 16:345, 1979.

Coggins, C.H.: Renal failure in lymphoma. *Kidney Int.* 17:847, 1980.

Cohen, A.H., and Border, W.A.: Myeloma kidney. An immunomorphogenetic study of renal biopsies. *Lab. Invest.* 42:248, 1980.

Finkel, P.N., Kronenberg, K., Pesce, A.J., et al.: Adult Fanconi syndrome, amyloidosis and marked K-light chain proteinuria. *Nephron* 10:1, 1973.

Ganeval, D., Mignon, F., Preud'homme, J-L., et al.: Visceral deposition of monoclonal light chains and immunoglobulins: A study of renal and immunopathologic abnormalities. *Adv. Nephrol.* 11:25, 1982.

Ganeval, D., Noël, L-H., Preud'homme, J-L., Droz, D. and Grünfeld, J-P.: Light-chain deposition disease: Its relation with AL-type amyloidosis (Editorial review). *Kidney Int.* 26:1, 1984.

Nicogossian, A., Lin, C.S., Mailloux, L.U., et al.: Diffuse lymphosarcoma of the kidneys manifested solely as progressive azotemia. *Mt. Sinai J. Med. N.Y.* 39:383, 1972.

Papadimitriou, J.M., and Matz, L.R.: The origin of multinucleated giant cells in myeloma kidney from mononuclear phagocytes. An ultrastructural study. *Pathology* 11:583, 1979.

Pascal, R.R.: Renal manifestations of extrarenal neoplasms. *Hum. Pathol.* 11:7, 1980.

Randolph, V.L., Hall, W., and Bramson, W.: Renal failure due to lymphomatous infiltration of the kidneys. *Cancer* 52:1120, 1983.

Silva, F.G., Pirani, C.L., Mesa-Tejada, R., et al.: The kidneys in plasma cell dyscrasias. A review and a clinicopathologic study of 50 patients. In Fenoglio, C., and Wolff, M. (Eds.): *Progress in Surgical Pathology.* New York: Masson Publishing, 1982, vol. 5, pp. 131–175.

Tubbs, R.R., Gephardt, G.N., McMahon, J.T., et al.: Light chain nephropathy. *Amer. J. Med.* 71:263, 1981.

Weiss, J.H., Williams, R.H., Galla, J.H., et al.: Pathophysiology of acute Bence-Jones protein nephrotoxicity in the rat. *Kidney Int.* 20:198, 1981.

Chapter 13

Chung-Park, M., Ricanati, E., Lankerani, M., et al.: Case reports: Acquired renal cysts and multiple renal cell and urothelial tumors. *Amer. Soc. Clin. Pathol.* 79:238, 1982.

Faraggiana, T., and Grishman, E.: Loss of podocyte cell coat in acute renal failure associated with massive proteinuria. *Fed. Proc. Fed. Amer. Soc. Exp. Biol.* 42:523, 1983.

McManus, J.F.A., and Hughson, M.D.: New therapies and new pathologies: End-stage dialysis kidneys. *Arch. Pathol. Lab. Med.* 103:53, 1979.

McManus, J.F.A., Hughson, M.D., Henniger, G.R., et al.: Dialysis enhances renal epithelial proliferations. *Arch. Pathol. Lab. Med.* 104:192, 1980.

Mihatsch, M.J., Torhorst, J., Straumann, U., et al.: Inter-

REFERENCES

stitial nephritis accompanying glomerulonephritis: Frequency, morphology, functional and prognostic significance. *Kidney Int.* 20:140, 1981.

Chapter 14

Austwick, P.K.C., Carter, R.L., Greig, J.B., et al.: Balkan (endemic) nephropathy. *Contrib. Nephrol.* 16:154, 1979.

Bolton, W.K., Atuk, N.O., Rametta, C., et al.: Reversible renal failure from isolated granulomatous renal sarcoid. *Clin. Nephrol.* 5:88, 1976.

Churg, J., and Madrazo, A.: Radiation nephritis. *Perspect. Nephrol. Hypertension* 6:83, 1977.

Dobrin, R.S., Vernier, R.L., and Fish, A.J.: Acute eosinophilic interstitial nephritis and renal failure with bone marrow-lymph node granulomas and anterior uveitis: A new syndrome. *Amer. J. Med.* 59:325, 1975.

Graber, M.L., Cogan, M.G., and Connor, D.G.: Idiopathic acute interstitial nephritis. *West. J. Med.* 129:72, 1978.

Hall, P.W., III, and Dammin, G.J.: Balkan nephropathy. *Nephron* 22:281, 1978.

Keane, W.F., Crosson, J.T., Staley, N.A., et al.: Radiation-induced renal disease: A clinicopathologic study. *Amer. J. Med.* 60:127, 1976.

Luxton, R.W.: Radiation nephritis: A long-term study of fifty-four patients. *Lancet* 2:1221, 1961.

Madrazo, A., Suzuki, Y., and Churg, J.: Radiation nephritis: Acute changes following high doses of radiation. *Amer. J. Pathol.* 54:507, 1969.

Madrazo, A., Suzuki, Y., and Churg, J.: Radiation nephritis: II. Chronic changes after high doses of radiation. *Amer. J. Pathol.* 61:37, 1970.

Muther, R.S., McCarron, D.A., and Bennett, W.M.: Renal manifestations of sarcoidosis. *Arch. Intern. Med.* 141:643, 1981.

Sattler, T.A., Dimitrov, T., and Hall, P.W.: Relation between endemic (Balkan) nephropathy and urinary-tract tumors. *Lancet* 1:278, 1977.

INDEX

Page numbers in bold type refer to extensive discussion or illustrations.

Abortion, septic, 136
Abscess, 21, 22, 34
Acetaminophen, 59
Acetylsalicylic acid, 56, 59
Acidosis, metabolic, 56
Actinomyces, 22
Acute Tubular Injury/necrosis (ATN), 22, 136, 138
  – – –, hemoglobinuric, **139, 142, 144**
  – – –, ischemic (vasomotor nephropathy), **138, 140, 142, 154**
  – – –, myoglobinuric, **139, 144**
  – – –, nephrotoxic, 136, **137**, 138, **140, 146, 148, 150, 152**
  – – –, post-renal, 136
  – – –, pre-renal, 136
  – – –, renal, 136
  – – –, toxic, 136, **140**
Adenovirus, 22
Adriamycin, 59
Aedes aegypti mosquito, transmitter of epidemic hemorrhagic fever, 36
Alcohol, as a cause of myoglobinuria, 139
Allergic reaction, drug induced, 55
Alloantigen, 78
Allograft, renal, *See* Renal allograft
Allopurinol, 59, 82, 83
Alport's Syndrome, *See* Syndrome
Amikacin, 59
Aminoaciduria, 78, 80, 120, 185
Aminoglycoside, 59, 137
Amphotericin B, 59
Ampicillin, 59, 83
Amyloid deposits, 185, 186
Amyloidosis, renal, 36
  –, secondary, 186
Analgesic abuse, 56, 57
  –, nephropathy, *See* Nephropathy, analgesic
Anomaly, urinary tract, 23
  –, vesicoureteric junction, 23
Anti-basement membrane disease, 77
  – – –, anti-GBM, 78
  – – –, anti-TBM, 77
Antibiotics, 55, 137
Antibody
  –, allo-, 77, 78
  –, anti-TBM, 77, 78, 83
  –, auto-, 77, 78
Aortic valve prosthesis, 121
Arsenic, 137
Arsine, 137, 139
Arteriosclerosis, 119

Arteritis, 137
Ask- Upmark kidney, 23, 95
Aspergillus, 22
Aspirin, 56
Autoradiography, 118
Azathioprine, 59, 83

Bacilli, acid-fast, 35
  –, alcohol-fast, 35
Bacitracin, 59
Bacterial endocarditis, 79
  –, infection, 34, 35, 81
  –, pyelonephritis, acute, 21
  –, chronic, 23
Basement membrane thickening, 57, 186
  – –, disruption, 56, 81, 138
Bence-Jones protein, 184, 185, 186
Bile nephrosis, **172**
Bismuth, 59, 118, **130,** 137
Blackwater fever, 139
Bladder, neuropathic, 24
Blastomycetes, 22
Blood transfusion, incompatible, 3, 139
Boric acid, 59
Brucellosis, 2
Busulfan, 59

Cadmium, 120
Calcification, 109, 119, 120
Calcium deposits, 158
  –, elevated levels in serum, 157
  –, versinate, 59
Calculi, renal, 25, 34, 160, 200
Calices, clubbed, 24, 94
  –, deformed, 24, 34, 95
  –, dilated, 24, 34, 93
Cancer, breakdown of cells, 158
Candida infection, 22
Capillary sclerosis, 57
Capreomycin, 59
Carbenicillin, 59, 83
Carbimazole, 59
Carbon tetrachloride, 137
Carcinoma, 186
  –, in analgesic nephropathy, 57, 66
  –, in Balkan nephropathy, 199
  –, in a cyst, end stage kidney, 193
  –, in lead nephropathy, 118
  –, renal cell, 34
  –, transitional cell, 57, 199
Cast, pigmented, 139
  –, tubular, 138, 185

CCNU (chloroethyl-cyclohexyl nitrosourea), 2, 58
Cell mediated hypersensitivity, 81
Cephalexine, 59, 83
Cephaloridine, 59
Cephalosporines, 137
Cephalothin, 59, 83
Chloramphenicol, 59
Chloroquine, 55
Cisplatin, 59, 119, 120, 137
Clofibrate, 59
Cloxacillin, 78
Colistin, 59
Collecting duct, 5
Complement, C3, granular deposit, 80
 – –, linear deposit, 78, 83
Conn's syndrome, *See* Syndrome
Copper, 121, 126
Corticosteroid, 55
Co-trimoxazole, 59, 83
Crush injury, 136, 139
Cryoglobulin, 186
Cryoglobulinemia, mixed, 3, **79,** 186
Cryptococcus infection, 22
Crystalluria, sulfonamides, 137
Crystals, oxalates, 137, 160, 193
 –, protein, in multiple myeloma, 185
 –, urates, 159
Cyclosporine, 59
Cystinosis, 3, 160
Cystitis, acute hemorrhagic, 22
 –, tuberculous, 35
Cytomegalovirus, 22

Degranulated basophils, 82
 –, eosinophils, 82
Dehydration in infants, 108, 109
Dengue fever, 35, 36
Dextran, 161
Diabetes insipidus, nephrogenic, 57, 80
 –, mellitus, 34, 108, 109
Dialysis, long term, 24, 193
Diethylene glycol, 137
Diflunisal, 59
Dilatation, diffuse pelvicaliceal, 25
 –, ureteric, 25
Dimethoxyphenylpenicilloyl, 83
Dimethylchlortetracyclin, 59
Dioxane, 137
Diphtheria, 2, 22
Discoloration, brownish, in analgesic
 papillary necrosis, 57
DNA products, 79
Drug-induced hypersensitivity, 55, 81, 82
Drugs, anticancer, 58, 119
Dysplasia, renal, 23, 94

E. coli, 21
EDTA, 118

Endarteritis, disuse, 193
Endocarditis, bacterial, 79
End-stage kidney, **193, 194, 196**
Eosinophilia, blood, 55, 82
 – –, transient, 82
 –, tissue, 56
Epidemic hemorrhagic fever, 2, 35, **36, 37, 46**
Ethylene glycol, 137, 160

Fanconi's syndrome, *See* Syndrome
Fatty change (degeneration), **170, 182**
Fenoprofen, 59, 82, 83
Fetal anoxia as a cause of hemorrhagic
 papillary necrosis, 109
Foam cells, 34
Fungemia, 22
Fungus infection, 21, 22
Furosemide, 59, 82, 83

Gentamicin, 59
Giant cell, 78, 82, 159
 – –, histiocytic, 34
 – –, multinucleated, 35, 185
Glafenine, 59, 83
Glomerular basement membrane, 78
Glomerular diseases, **192, 194**
Glomeruli in acute tubular necrosis, 138
Glomerulonephritis
 –, anti-GBM, 78
 –, bacterial immune complex, **79**
 –, hypocomplementemic, **80, 86, 90**
 –, immune complex, 78
 – – –, in leprosy, 36
 – – –, in syphilis, 36
 –, membranous, 78, 119
 –, mixed cryoglubulinemia, 79
 –, post-streptococcal, 78
 –, proliferative, 192
 –, Sjögren's syndrome, 79
 –, SLE, 79
Glomerulosclerosis, focal, 24, 57, 95
Glycogen deposition, **170**
Glycolate in oxalosis, 160
Glycols, 137
Glycosuria, 78, 79, 120
Glyoxalate in oxalosis, 160
Gold, 120
Goodpasture's disease, *See* Syndrome
Gout, 158
 –, granuloma, 159
 –, secondary, 158
Granuloma, 34
 –, drug induced, 56
 –, in IgE-type hypersensitivity, 82
 –, in myeloma kidney, 185
 –, necrotizing, 35
 –, sarcoid, 157, 200
 –, tuberculous, 35

Heavy metals, 2, **118,** 136, 137
Hemochromatosis, 121
Hemoglobinuria, 121, 137, 139
 –, paroxysmal, 139
Hemolytic anemia, 121
Hemorrhagic fever, 36
Hemosiderin, 121
Hemosiderosis, 121
Histoplasma, 22
Hyaline droplet degeneration, **170**
Hydronephrosis, 2, 93, 94, **96, 98**
 –, secondary, 35
Hyperaldosteronism, secondary, 161
Hypercalcemia, 157, 200
 –, idiopathic, 157
Hypercalciuria, 157
Hypergammaglobulinemia in plasma cell
 dyscrasias, 184
Hyperglobulin M-type of immunodeficiency,
 22
Hyperlipemia, 192
Hypernatremia, 137
Hyperoxaluria, primary, 160
 –, secondary, 160
Hyperparathyroidism, 157
 –, primary, 157
 –, secondary, 157
Hypersensitivity, 81
 –, cell mediated, 81
 –, drug, 55, 83
 –, IgE type, 82
 –, immediate reaction, 83
 –, lymphocyte, 81
Hypertension, 95, 118
Hyperthyroidism, 157
Hyperuricemia, 158
Hypocomplementemia, 80
Hypokalemia, 55, 161
Hypoplasia, segmental, *See* Segmental
 hypoplasia

IgE, 82, 83
IgG, granular deposits, 80
 –, linear deposits, 78, 83
IgM, granular deposits, 80
Immune complex diseases, 2, 79, 80
Immunoblast, 80
Immunoglobulins, 184
 –, light chains, 120, 185
Immunosupression, 80
Inclusion bodies, lead, 118
 – –, myeloma, 185, 186
Incompatible blood transfusion, 139
Indomethacin, 59
Infection, renal, 2, **21ff**, 26
 – –, special forms, **34ff**
 – –, specific, 21, **35ff**
Interstitial nephritis, 36
 – –, acute, 22, 138

 – –, chronic, 21, 57
 – –, focal, 22
 – –, megalocytic, 2, 35
Interstitial renal edema, 36, 56
Interstitium, normal, **5,** 6, **20**
Intrarenal reflux (IRR), **23,** 24, 25, 94
Intrauterine asphyxia, 109
Iodinated radiographic contrast media, 137
Iron, 121, 172
Ischemia, 138, 193
 –, pre-transplant, 80
Isosthenuria, 137

Jaundice, 108

Kanamycin, 59
Kidney, end stage, 193
 –, myeloma, *See* Myeloma kidney
 –, scarred, 24

Lead, 118
 –, in gouty nephropathy, 159
 –, inclusions, stains for, **118**
Legionnaire's disease, 2, 22
Leprosy, 2, 21, **35, 36, 46,** 81
 –, amyloidosis, 36
 –, glomerulonephritis, 36
 –, lepromatous, 36
Leptospirosis, 22
Lesch-Nyhan Syndrome, *See* Syndrome
Leukemia, 3, 158
Leukemic infiltration, **187, 188**
Leukocyturia, sterile, 56
Light chain, 184, 185, 186
 – –, nephropathy, *See* Nephropathy, light
 chain
Lipiduria, 192
Lithium, 57
Lobal nephronia, acute, 22
Loop of Henle, 5
Lupus Erythematosus, *See* Systemic lupus
 erythematosus
Lymphoid follicle formation, 24, 25
Lymphokines, 83
Lymphoma, 3, 158
Lymphomatous infiltration, **187**
Lymphoproliferative neoplastic disease, 186

Macrophage, 34, 35, 185
Malacoplakia, 2, **34,** 35, **40, 53, 54**
Malaria, 139
Maldevelopment, congenital, 23, 94
Maldifferentiation, 23, 94
Malignant lesions as a cause of light-chain
 nephropathy, 186
Manic-depressive psychosis, 57
Mannitol, 161
McArdle's disease, 139
Measles, 81

Medullary cavities in analgesic nephropathy, 56, 109
Medullary cystic disease, 184
Megalocytic interstitial nephritis, 2, **35, 42**
Melanuria, **172**
6-Mercaptopurin, 59
Mercurial diuretics, 137
Mercurials, 59
Mercury, 119, 120, 137
Mesangial cell proliferation, 36
  – sclerosis, 36, 120
  – widening, 120
Metabolic disorders, **157ff**
Metaplastic bone and cartilage in end stage kidney, 193
Methemoglobin, 139
Methicillin, 56, 59, 78, 82, 83
Methotrexate, 59
Methoxyflurane, 160
Methylphenidate, 59
Michaelis-Guttman bodies, 35
B₂ Microglobulin, 120
Milk alkali syndrome, *See* Syndrome
Minocycline, 59
Mixed IgG-IgM cryoglobulinemia, *See* Cryoglobulinemia, mixed
Monilia, 22
Monocytes, 34
Mucor, 22
Multiple Sclerosis, 93
Mycobacteria, 35
  –, leprae, 35
Myelin figures, 34
Myeloma, multiple, 138, 158, 184, 186
  –, kidney, 3, **184, 185, 188**
Myeloproliferative disorders, 158
Myoglobin, 139
Myoglobinuria, 2, **139**

Nafcillin, 59, 83
Naproxen, 59, 83
Necrosis in situ of papilla, 56
  –, papillary, *See* Papillary necrosis
  –, tubular, *See* Tubular necrosis
Neoplastic lytic lesions, 158
Nephritis, *See also* tubulo-interstitial nephritis
  –, acute interstitial, in systemic infection, 21, **22**
  –, acute lymphomatous, 22
  –, anti GBM and anti TBM, 78
  –, epidemica, 36
  –, radiation, 3, **199, 202, 206**
  –, scarlatinal, 22
Nephrocalcinosis, 157, 158, **174, 176, 178**, 200
Nephropathy, acute vasomotor, 138
  –, analgesic, 2, 23, **56ff**, 57, **62, 64, 66, 72, 74, 108, 109**

  –, –, pathology, 56, 57, 109
  –, –, radiology, 56
  –, Balkan endemic, 3, **199, 200, 202**
  –, bile, 3, **172**
  –, cadmium, **120**
  –, cisplatin, **119, 126**
  –, copper, 3, **121, 126**
  –, cystinosis, 3, 160
  –, fatty, 3
  –, gold, **120**
  –, glycogen, 3
  –, gouty, 158, 159
  –, heavy metal induced, **118ff**, 120
  –, hemoglobinuric, **139**
  –, hyaline droplet, 3, 170
  –, hypercalcemic, 3, **157, 158, 162, 164, 176, 178**
  –, hypokalemic, 3, **160, 161, 168, 182**
  –, iron, 3, **121, 172**
  –, lead, **118, 122, 128, 130**
  –, light chain, 3, **185, 186, 188, 190**
  –, lithium, 2, **57, 66, 74**
  –, mercury, **119, 124, 132**
  –, myoglobinuric, **139**
  –, nitrosourea (CCNU), 2, **58**
  –, osmotic, 3, **170**
  –, oxalate, 3, **159, 160, 166, 168, 178, 180**
  –, reflux, *See* Reflux nephropathy
  –, sarcoid granulomatous, 3, **200, 202, 204**
  –, silver, **121, 134**
  –, sodium losing, 82
  –, urate, 3, **158, 159, 164, 166**
  –, –, acute, 159
  –, –, chronic, 158
  –, vasomotor, 136, 138
Nephrotic syndrome, 36, 78, 82, 119, 120, 186, 192
Nitrosourea, *See* Nephropathy, nitrosourea
Nocardia, 22

Obstructive uropathy, 2, 25, **93ff, 96, 98**, 108
Oral contraception, 95
Oxacillin, 59, 83
Oxalate, 160
  –, calcium, 160
  – crystals, 137, 160, 193
Oxalosis, 160
Oxyhemoglobin, 139

Papillae, compound, 23
  –, conical, 23
Papillary necrosis, 2, 21, 22, 56, 57, 94, **108, 109**, 136
  – –, advanced, 57
  – –, in amyloidosis, **114**
  – –, in analgesic nephropathy, 56, **108, 109**
  – –, in diabetes mellitus, **108, 109, 110**
  – –, hemorrhagic, in newborns, 109, 112

Papillary necrosis, (*continued*)
– –, non-infectious, acute, 23
– –, in obstructive uropathy, 94, **108, 109**
– –, in sickle cell disease, **110, 116**
– –, in vascular diseases, **112, 114**
– –, in vascular diseases, **112, 114**
Para-amino salicylic acid, 59
Paranomycin, 59
Paraplegia, 93
Parasitic infections (infestation), 22, 35, 37, 81
Penicillin, 59, 82, 83
Periglomerular fibrosis, 35
Phagolysosome, 34, 35, 138, 186
Phenacetin, 56
Phenazone, 59, 83
Phenindione, 59, 82, 83
Phenobarbital, 59, 83
Phenylbutazone, 59, 83
Phenytoin, 59, 83
Plasma cell, dyscrasia, 3, **184ff, 188**
– –, immature, 185
– –, leukemia, 184
– –, monoclonal, 184
Plasmacytoma, soft tissue, 184
Plumbism, chronic, 118
Polycytemia vera, 158
Polymyxin B, 59
Polyomavirus, 22
Posterior urethral valve, 23, 94
Pregnancy, 95
Premature infant, 109
Prolonged labor, 109
Proteus mirabilis, 34
Pyelitis, 21
Pyelonephritis, 2, 108
–, acute, 2, **21ff,** 136
–, –, bacterial, 2, **21ff, 26**
–, chronic, 2, 23, 25, **30, 32**
–, –, bacterial, 23
– – , non obstructive, **23**
–, –, obstructive, 2, **25**
–, –, –, pathology, 24
–, –, –, reflux associated, 23
–, fungal, 22
–, obstructive focal, 185
–, special forms, **34ff**
–, tuberculous, 35
–, viral, 22
–, xanthogranulomatous, 2, 25, **34, 38, 48, 50, 51, 52**
Pyonephrosis, **2,** 94, **98**
–, tuberculous, 35
Pyridoxine deficiency, 160

Quinine, 139

Radiation nephritis, *See* Nephritis, radiation
Radiographic contrast media, 137

Reflux, intrarenal, *See* Intrarenal reflux
–, sterile, 94
Reflux nephropathy, 2, 21, 23, **24**, 25, **94, 95, 98, 100, 102, 104, 106**
– –, acute experimental, 22
– –, focal, 94
– –, generalized, 94
– –, pathology, 24
– –, radiology, 24
Renal allograft, **78, 80, 84**
Renal failure, acute (ARF), 35, 57, 108, 119, 121, 136, 139, 185
– – –, hemoglobinuric, **139, 142, 144**
– – –, myoglobinuric, **139, 144**
– – –, nephrotoxic, 136, **137,** 138, **140, 146, 148**
– – –, postrenal, 136
– – –, prerenal, 136
– – –, renal, 136
– – –, vasomotor, **138, 140, 142, 150, 152, 154**
Renal insufficiency, (failure), chronic, 55, 120, 158
Renal transplant in oxalosis, 160
Renal tubular acidosis, 78, 80
– – –, distal, 82
Renal vein thrombosis, 109
Rheumatoid arthritis, 120
Rifampicin, 59, 82, 83

Sarcoidosis, 157, **200, 202, 204**
Scarlet fever, 22
Scarring, corticomedullary, 24
–, renal, 25
Schaumann bodies, 200
Segmental hypoplasia, 23, 95
Septic abortion, *See* Abortion, septic
Shock, 136
Sickle cell disease, 23, 110, 116, 121
Silver, 121
Sjögren syndrome, *See* Syndrome
Skin exanthema (rash), 55, 82
Snake venom, 139
Solvents, 136, 137
Spina bifida, 93
Stain, hematoxylin and eosin for calcium, 158
–, for myeloma inclusions, 185
–, periodic acid-Schiff (PAS), 34, 35, 57
–, phosphotungstic acid hematoxylin, 185
–, rubeanic acid for copper, 121
–, Ziel-Neelson, 35
Stones, renal, 25, 34, 160, 200
– –, urate, 159
Streptococcus, 2
–, group A, 22
Streptomycin, 59
Sulfonamides, 56, 59, 82, 83, 137

Syndrome, Alport's, 184, 192
–, Conn's, 161
–, Fanconi's, 79, 119, 185
–, Goodpasture's, **78**
–, Lesch-Nyhan, 158
–, milk-alkali, 157
–, Sjögren's, **79, 80, 86, 92**
Syphilis, 2, **36,** 118
Systemic lupus erythematosus (SLE), **79, 84, 86, 88, 89,** 192

T cell, 83
Tamm-Horsfall protein, 93, 138, 185
Test, Kveim, 200
–, tuberculin, 200
Tetracylcine, 55
Thiazides, 59, 82, 83
Thyroidization, 24
Tobramycin, 59
Tolmetin, 59
Tophus, 158
Toxoplasmosis, 2, 22
Transplant rejection, cellular type, 80
– –, vascular type, 81
Tuberculosis, 2, 21, **35, 44,** 81
–, miliary, 35
Tubular necrosis, acute, 2, 119, 120, **136**
– –, ischemic, 2, 136, **138**
– –, nephrotoxic, 136, **137,** 138
Tubulotoxic injury, acute, drug induced, 55, **60, 68, 70**
Tubule, collecting, 5, **16, 18**
–, distal, 5, **14, 16**
–, Henle's loop, 5, **14**
–, normal, **5ff**
–, proximal, 5, **6, 8, 10, 12**
Tubulo-interstitial disorders, (hereditary), 3, 184
Tubulo-interstitial lesions in glomerular and vascular diseases, 3, 192
Tubulo-interstitial Nephritis (TIN), 2, 21, **22,** 80, 81, 193
– – –, acute, 2, 36, 79
– – – –, bacterial, 2, **21ff, 26,** 109
– – – –, drug induced, 2, **55ff,** 78
– – – –, – –, hypersensitivity, 2, 22, **55, 60, 62**
– – – –, – –, IgE type, 2, **82, 83, 86**
– – – –, eosinophilic, **200, 201, 204**
– – – –, idiopathic, 3, 200
– – – –, infectious, **26**
– – –, associated with immune disorders, 2, **77ff, 84**
– – – –, antitubular basement membrane, 2, **77ff**
– – – –, cell mediated, 2, **81**
– – –, chronic, 21, 79, 119
– – – –, drug induced, 2, **56ff**
– – – –, idiopathic, 3, **201**
– – – –, infectious, 2, **23ff, 30, 32**
– – – –, non-obstructive, **23ff**
– – –, fungal, 2, **22, 28**
– – –, in glomerular diseases, **192**
– – –, hereditary, 184
– – –, hypersensitivity cell mediated, **81**
– – –, idiopathic, 3, 78, **200, 201**
– – – –, granulomatous, 3, **201, 204**
– – –, immune complex, 2, **79ff, 84**
– – –, immunologically-mediated, 77
– – –, – –, classification, 77
– – –, in neoplastic disorders, **184ff**
– – –, recurrent, drug induced, 55
– – –, in vascular diseases, 192, 193
– – –, viral, 2, **22, 28, 30**
– – –, with systemic infection, 2, 22
Tubulo-interstitial nephropathy associated with metabolic disorders, 3, **157ff**
– – –, associated with neoplastic disorders, 3, **184**
Tubulorrhexis, 56, 138

Uranyl, 137
Urate, ammonium, 159
–, granuloma, 158
–, gravel formation, 159
–, overload, acute, 158
–, sodium, 159
Ureteral ectopia, 94
– obstruction, 22
– orifice, 23
Urethral stricture, 93
Uric acid, 159
– –, infarct, 159
Urinary tract obstruction, 25, 93
Urographic contrast media, 59
Uropathy, obstructive, *See* Obstructive uropathy
Urticaria, 80

Vacuolar change, **170**
Vancomycin, 59
Vasculitis, cutaneous, 80
–, renal, 56
Vasomotor nephropathy, *See* Acute tubular injury/necrosis
Vesico-ureteral reflux (VUR), 2, 21, **23,** 24, 25, 94
– – –, focal, 94
– – –, generalized, 94
– – –, secondary, 94
Viomycin, 59
Virus, 2, 21, 22, 36, 81
–, adeno, 22
–, arbo, 36
–, cytomegalo, 22
–, polyoma, BK-type, 22

Virus (*continued*)
 –, porcine corona, 200
Vitamin B$_6$ deficiency, 160
Vitamin D overdosage, 157

Waldenström's macroglobulinemia, 3, 184,
 186
Wegener's granulomatosis, 192
Wilson's disease, 3